Lip Diagnostics

Lip Diagnostics

New Reflection Zones of the Human Organs on the Lips

Dr. George Zdravkov

Author of
Qigong Hand Diagnostics

Copyright © 2019 by Dr. George Zdravkov

All rights reserved. This work may not be translated or copied in whole or in part without the written permission of the author except for brief excerpts in connection with reviews or scholarly analysis. Use in connection with any form of information storage and retrieval, electronic adaptation, computer software, or by similar or dissimilar methodology now known or hereafter developed is forbidden.

The use in this publication of trade names, trademarks, service marks and similar terms, even if they are not identified as such, is not to be taken as an expression of opinion as to whether or not they are subject to proprietary rights. The Publisher is not associated with any product mentioned in this book.

This publication is designed to provide accurate and authoritative information in regard to the subject matter covered at the time of publication. It is sold on the understanding that the Publisher is not engaged in rendering professional services. If professional advice or other expert assistance is required regarding any subject matter covered in this book, the services of a competent professional should be sought.

ISBN-13: 9781795706063

Printed in the United States of America

Cover design by David Julian
Author photograph by Nely Piper
Interior design by Ghislain Viau

CONTENTS

I.	Introduction	1
II.	Anatomical Characteristics of the Human Lips	9
III.	Reflection Zones of the Human Organs on the Lips	13
IV.	Pathological Changes in the Lips	15
V.	Manifestations of Pathologic Processes on the Lips	19
VI.	Manifestations of the Diseases on the Lip Organ Zones	31
	1. Pathologic Processes of the Pulmonary System	31
	1.1. Infections of the Upper Respiratory System – nose, sinuses, pharynx	
	1.2. Infections of the Lower Respiratory System – bronchus, lung	
	1.3. Allergy of the Upper Respiratory System – nose, sinuses, pharynx	
	1.4. Allergy of the Lower Respiratory System – bronchus, lung	
	1.5. Proliferative Processes in the Lungs – replacing functional with connective tissue, and tumors	
	1.6. Toxic Influences on the Lungs	
	2. Pathologic Processes of the Cardiovascular System	45
	2.1. Hypertension	
	2.2. Hypotension	
	2.3. Arrhythmia	
	2.4. Heart Attack	
	2.5. Heart Insufficiency	
	2.6. Varicose Veins	
	2.7. Lymphadenitis	
	3. Pathologic Processes of the Gastrointestinal System	60
	3.1. Gastritis. Ulcer of the Stomach	
	3.2. Enteritis	

3.3.	Colitis	
3.4.	Hepatitis. Cirrhosis	
3.5.	Cholecystitis. Cholelithiasis	
4.	Pathologic Processes of the Urogenital System	84
4.1.	Cystitis. Prostatitis	
4.2.	Glomerulonephritis. Kidney insufficiency	
4.3.	Nephrolithiasis	
4.4.	Tumors of the Urogenital System	
5.	Pathologic Processes of the Endocrine System	91
5.1.	Struma. Hyperthyroidism. Hypothyroidism	
5.2.	Diabetes Mellitus	
5.3.	Infections and Tumors of the Uterus and Ovaries	
5.4.	Breast	
6.	Pathologic Processes of the Brain and Peripheral Nerve System	109
6.1.	Neuroses	
6.2.	Headache. Migraine	
6.3.	Tremors	
6.4	Paralyses	
6.5	Tumors of the Nerve System	
6.6	Eyes	
7.	Pathologic Processes of the Bone-Muscular System	124
7.1	Fractures. Traumas	
7.2	Arthrosoarthritis	
7.3	Osteochondrosis	
8.	Pathologic Processes of the Skin	135

VII.	Lip Therapy	139
VIII.	Literature	141
	Glossary of Medical Terms	143
	About the Author	151

SECTION I

INTRODUCTION

The idea of writing this book rose in my mind more than thirty years ago. However, taking care of my patients and work on other projects did not allow me to complete it sooner. My first article on the reflection zones of organs on the lips was presented as *Biologically Active Points and Zones on the Human Lips* at The World Congress of Chinese Traditional Medicine, in Belgrade, Serbia in 1989.

It is well known that many reflection zones corresponding to various human organs are located on the ears [1], hands, and feet [2], irises [3], tongue [4], teeth [5]. See Fig. 1 on next page.

The reflection zones are used not only for diagnostic purposes, but for therapy as well.

Fig. 1 Reflection zones of the human organs on the ears, hands, feet, tongue, teeth, and irises.

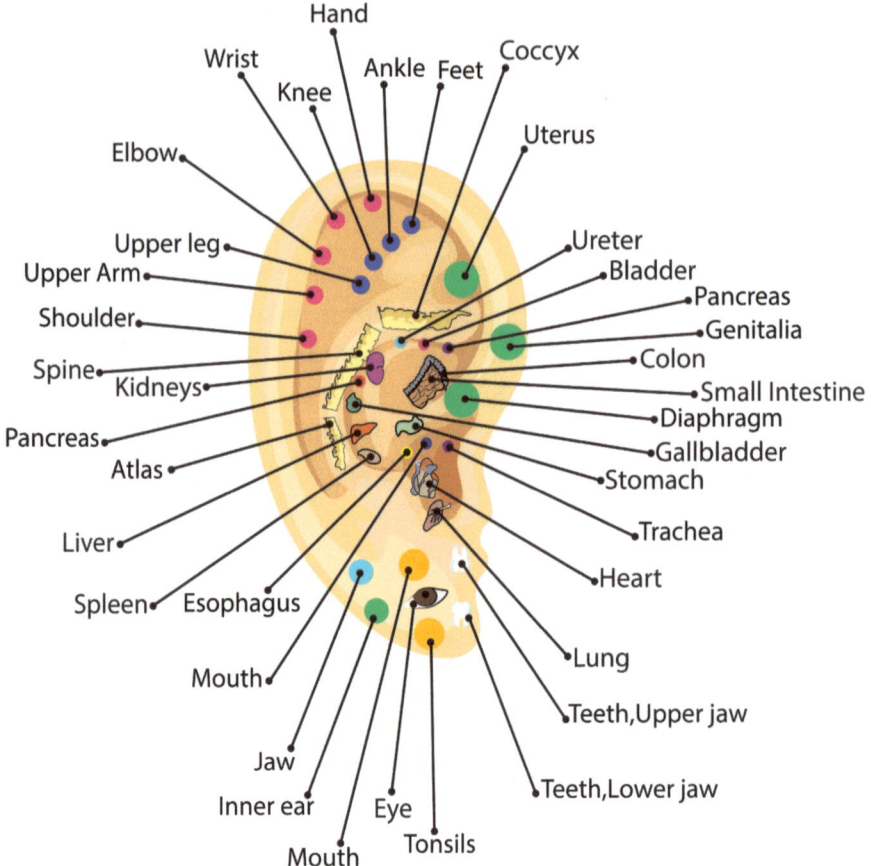

Reflection Zones on the Ears

New Reflection Zones of the Human Organs on the Lips

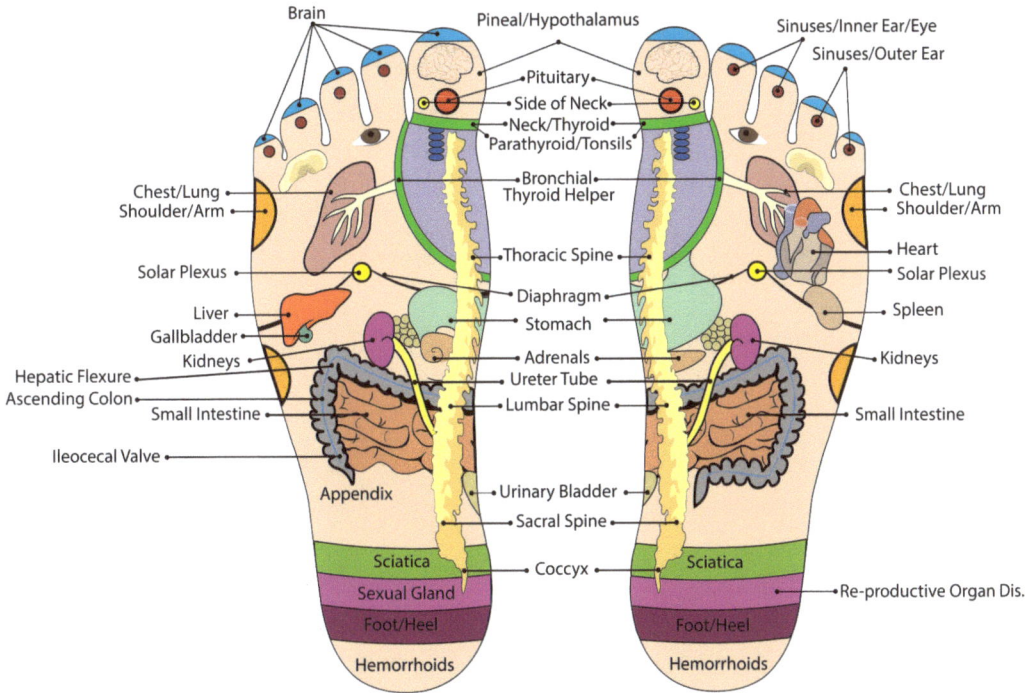

Reflection Zones on the Feet

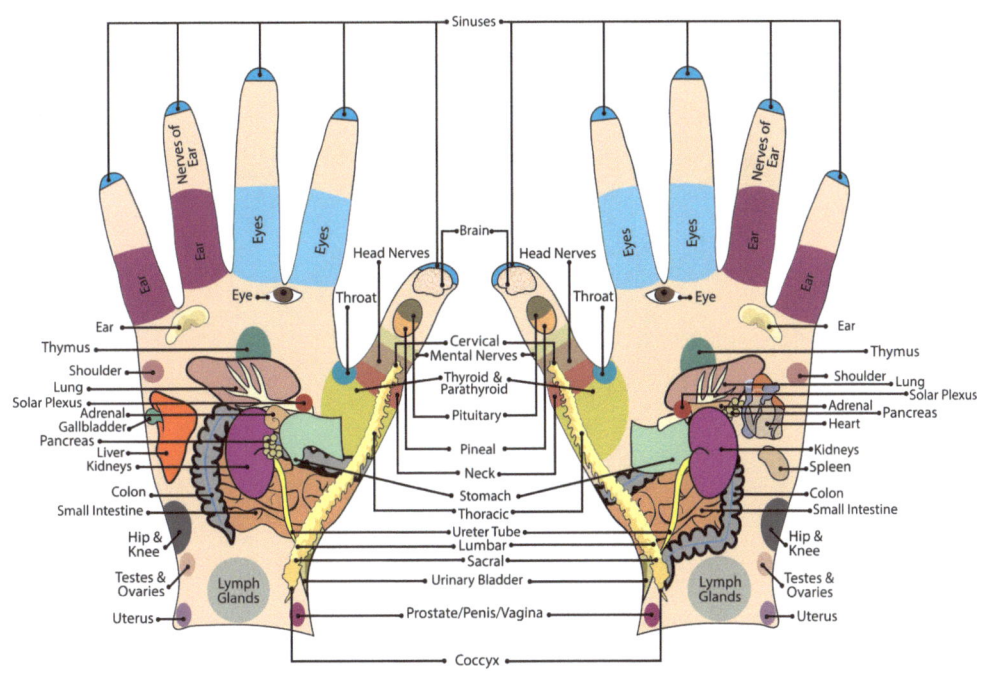

Reflection Zones on the Hands

Lip Diagnostics

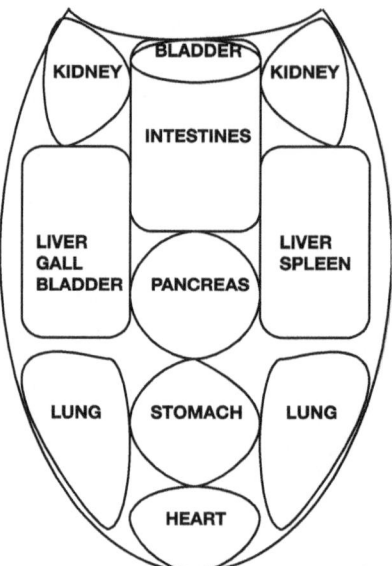

Reflection Zones on the Tongue

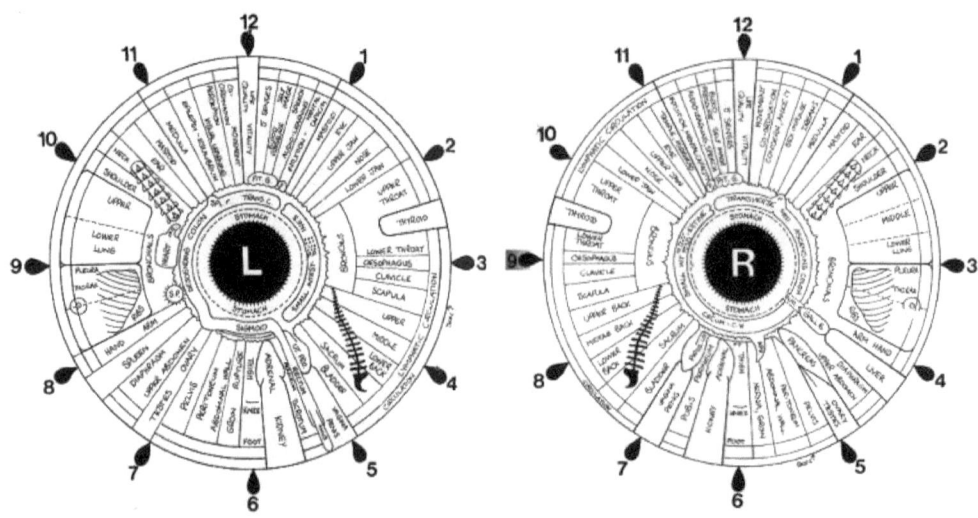

Reflection Zones on the Irises

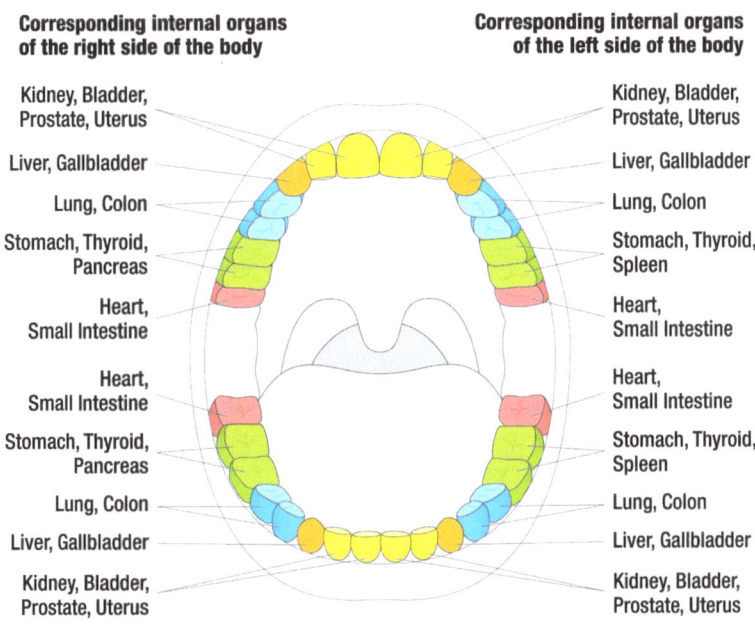

Reflexology Chart of the Teeth

Why are reflection zones of the organs on the lips so important?

The lips and the tops of the fingers are the most sensitive areas of the human body. They contain the greatest number of specialized sensory receptors in regard to the mechano-receptive somatic senses (tactile sensations, such as touch, pressure, vibration, tickling, and position sensations), thermoreceptive sensations (heat and cold) and pain. [6] The lips and finger tips have greater representation in somatosensory area I of the brain cortex than any other part of the body (localized in the postcentral gyrus of the human cerebral cortex – in Brodmann`s areas 3, 1 and 2) [6]. See Fig. 2 on next page.

Fig. 2. The Somatosensory Homunculus. Proportional Presentation of the Somatosensory Homunculus [7].

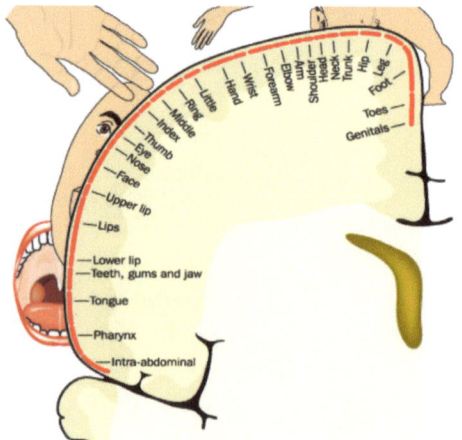
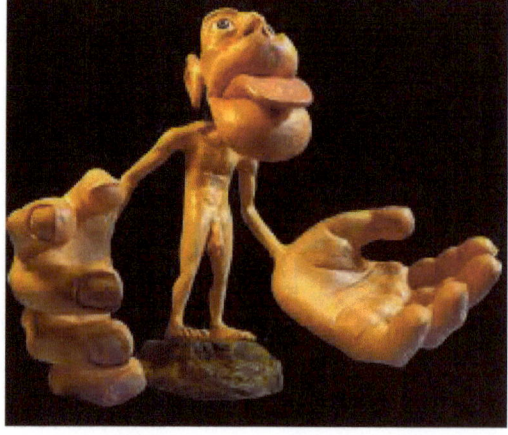

Somatosensory homunculus

Proportional presentation of the somatosensory homunculus

- When babies explore the world, every object they encounter is first brought to the lips. Each type of food and liquid is first examined in such a manner and is later recognized by lip memory.
- Touch sensation is the oldest type of existing sensation from an evolutionary point of view.
- The first thing that we do when experiencing pain or emotional stress is to unconsciously press together or bite the lips.
- Two of the most important energy channels in TCM, the Governing (Du mai, the Sea of Yang channel) and the Directing or Conception (Ren mai, the Sea of Yin channel) vessels reach the area of the lips. [8] These two channels control the function of, and carry information to, all organs and systems in the human body.

Fig. 3 Governing (Du mai, the Sea of Yang channel) and Directing or Conception (Ren mai, the Sea of Yin channel) Vessels.

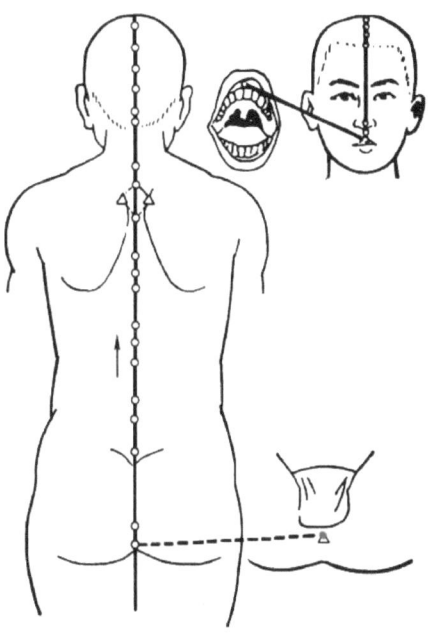

The Governing Channel (Du mai, the Sea of Yang channel) - GV

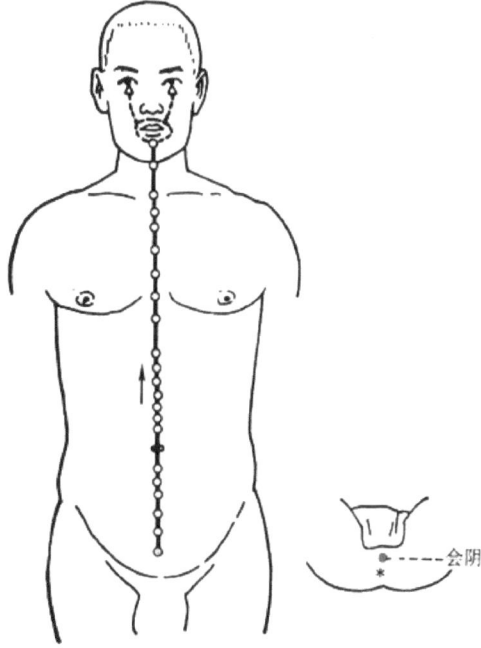

The Conception Channel (Ren mai, the Sea of Yin channel) - CV

SECTION II

FUNCTIONAL, ANATOMICAL, AND HISTOLOGICAL CHARACTERISTICS OF THE HUMAN LIPS

1. Functional Characteristics of the Human Lips

The lips are used for *eating functions*, holding, getting food into the mouth, and keeping out unwanted objects. The ability to make a narrow funnel with the lips in order to be able to perform a sucking motion is essential for babies in order to be able to breast-feed.

The lips are an important part of the speech apparatus in their *articulation function*. They are instrumental in the creation of different sounds – labial, bilabial, and labiodental, as well as vowel rounding.

Very high sensitivity to texture, warmth, and cold make the lips an important aid for babies and toddlers in terms of exploring unknown objects.

The lips are *an erogenous zone* and play a crucial role in kissing and other acts of intimacy. Estrogen levels have a very strong influence on facial structure (including fullness of the lips) during puberty and final maturation. The more estrogen a woman has, the larger her eyes, and the fuller her lips. These characteristics are perceived to be more feminine and thus more desirable from an evolutionary standpoint. [9]

The lips are included in our *facial expressions* and visibly express emotions such as a smile or a frown.

2. Anatomic and Histologic Characteristics of Human Lips

Human lips are constructed of the upper and lower lips, respectively the labium superior oris and labium inferior oris. [10] The lips are connected to the surrounding skin by the vermilion borders (see Fig. 4). The reddish area within the vermilion borders is named the vermilion zone. The vermilion border of the upper lip is known as the Cupid's bow. The protuberance located in the center of the upper lip is named the procheilon. The vertical groove from the procheilon to the nasal septum is called the philtrum. The upper lip covers the anterior surface of the body of the maxilla. The lower lip covers the anterior body of the mandible.

The muscles acting on the lips derive from the mesoderm of the second pharyngeal arch and are motor supplied by a facial nerve (7th cranial nerve). The muscles acting on the lips are the Buccinator and Orbicularis oris (a complex of muscles). The muscles included in lip elevation are Levator labii superior, Levator labii superioris alaeque nasi, Levator anguli oris, Zygomaticus major, and Zygomaticus minor. The muscles included in lip depression are the Risorius, Depressor anguli oris, Depressor labii inferioris, and Mentalis. [10]

Sensory nerve supply to the lips is provided by the trigeminal nerve (5th cranial nerve, maxillary and mandibular branches). The infraorbital nerve, a branch of the maxillary branch, supplies the upper lip and the skin of the face between the upper lip and the lower eyelid. The mental nerve, a branch of the mandibular branch (via the inferior alveolar nerve), supplies the skin and mucous membrane of the lower lip and gum. [10]

The superior and inferior labial branches of the facial artery, a branch of the external carotid artery, supply blood to the lips. [10]

The skin of the lips is comprised of stratified squamous epithelia. The skin of the lips is very thin (3-5 cellular layers) compared to typical facial skin (up to sixteen layers). The red color of the lips is due to the blood vessels below the thin epithelium. With light skin color, the skin of the lips contains fewer melanocytes (cells which produce the melanin pigment) and looks brighter and redder. With darker skin colors, the skin contains more melanin and looks darker. [10]

Fig. 4 Anatomic Characteristics of the Human Lips.

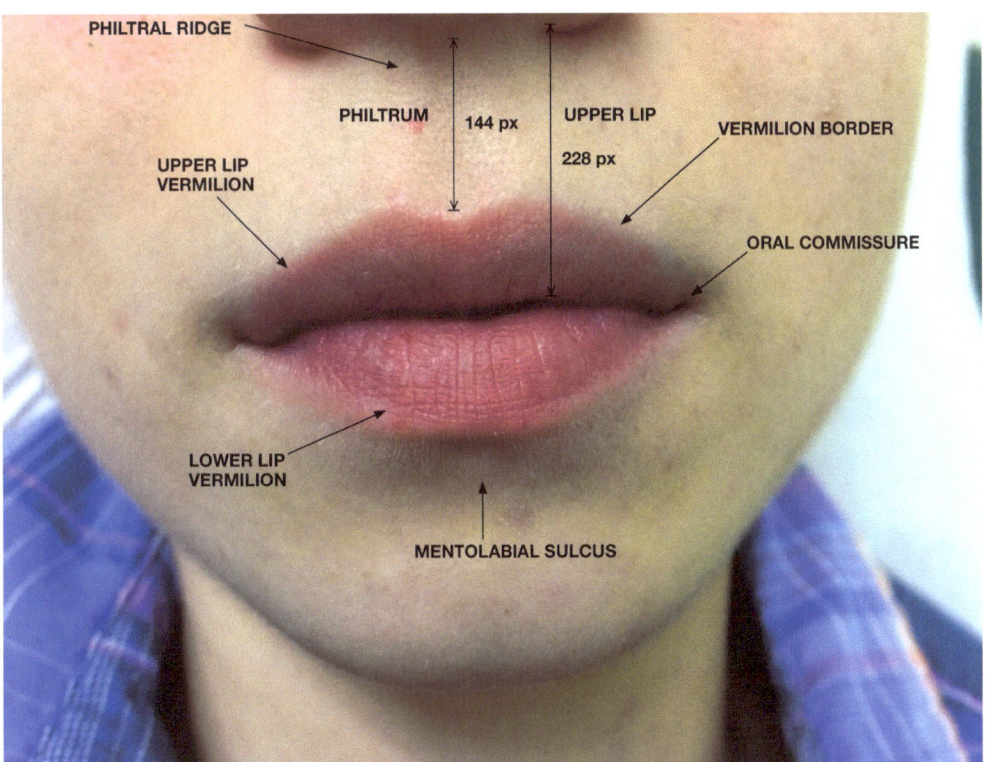

SECTION III
REFLECTION ZONES OF THE ORGANS ON THE LIPS

Fig. 5 presents the reflection zones of the organs on the lips. The upper lip includes the reflection zones of the organs above the diaphragm. The lower lip includes the reflection zones of the organs below the diaphragm. The vermilion border is a reflection of the skin. The right side of the lip contains the organs which are found on the left side of the body, and the left side of the lip contains the reflection of the organs found on the right side.

Pathologic processes with a very long history can show changes, not only in the lip organ zones, but also on the skin around the lips. The older the disease, the more changes can be seen in the lip reflection zone and surrounding skin. Many examples will be presented in the next chapters.

Fig. 5 Reflection zones of the human organs on the lips

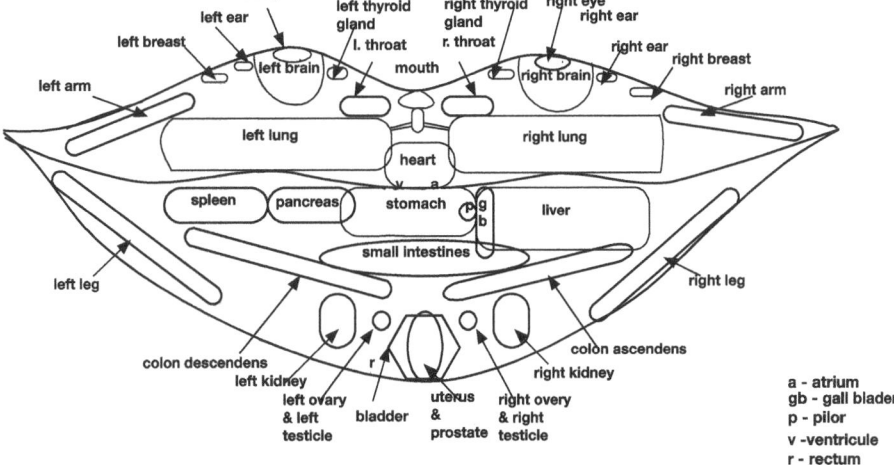

SECTION IV

PATHOLOGIC CHANGES AND DISEASES OF THE LIPS FROM THE PERSPECTIVE OF WESTERN AND EASTERN MEDICINE

This chapter will list the most frequent and important pathologic changes and diseases of the lips from both Western and Eastern Medical Traditions.

1. Diseases of the Lip in Western Medicine

Genetic Diseases:
- Cleft lip and cleft palate. Cleft lip and cleft palate are openings or splits in the upper lip, the roof of the mouth (palate), or both. Cleft lip and cleft palate result when the facial structures that are developing in an unborn baby do not close completely. Cleft lip and cleft palate are among the most common birth defects in humans. [11, 12]
- Hapsburg lip can be described as a thick, overdeveloped lower lip. [11, 12]
- Fetal alcohol syndrome is responsible for the thinning of the vermilion on the upper lip and the flattening of the philtrum.
- Double lip, is a redundant fold of tissue on the mucosal side of the upper lip that gives the appearance of a second lip and that may be accentuated by habitual sucking of the lip between the teeth.
- Lip pits (congenital lip fistulas) are congenital depressions, usually bilateral and symmetrically placed, on the vermilion portion of the lower lip. These pits may be circular or may be present as a transverse slit. The depression represents a blind fistula that penetrates downward into the lower lip to

a depth of 0.5 to 2.5 cm. They often exude viscid saliva on application of pressure. [13]

Neurologic Diseases

- Lip biting is an oral habit in which either lip is placed between the teeth with a more, or less, forcible application of the teeth to the lips.
- Lip droop is an unnatural condition where the lower lip hangs when it is not being used during pretension and mastication. This syndrome is accompanied by a lack of sensitivity. Unilateral droop is usually an indication of facial paralysis. Bilateral droop occurs in many conditions that fall under general paralysis, e.g. botulism.

Nutritional Deficits and Environmental Factors

- Dry, cracked lips have also been associated with a deficiency of certain B vitamins (B2, B12). For example, although it is not a typical symptom, cracked lips (especially at the corners) can sometimes signal a deficiency of folic acid. [14] Cracked lips can also be a symptom of a riboflavin (vitamin B2) deficiency. Those at risk for this condition include people who are elderly or have a chronic illness or alcohol dependence. A riboflavin deficiency can typically be remedied with a balanced, healthy diet or a vitamin supplement. [15] Dry, cracked, and inflamed lips can indicate iron insufficiency.
- Dry, cracked, or peeling lips can occur through overexposure to wind, sun, dry air, and dehydration.

Infectious Diseases

- Herpes simplex virus infection (HSV-1 type). Oral herpes is an infection caused by the herpes simplex virus. The virus causes painful sores on the lips, gums, tongue, roof of the mouth, and inside the cheeks. [16]
- Syphilis. During the first stage of infection, syphilis may appear as sores, known as chancres, on the lips, the tip of the tongue, the gums, or at the back of the mouth near the tonsils. Chancres start as small red patches and grow into larger, open sores that can be red, yellow, or gray in color. [17]
- Fungal or yeast infection. A fungal infection most commonly appears as cracking in the corners of the mouth, and is referred to as angular cheilitis. [18]
- Mucocele occur when a salivary gland is blocked by infections or trauma. A mucous cyst, also known as a mucocele, is a fluid-filled swelling that occurs on the *lips* or in the mouth. [19]

Allergic reactions
- Foods, beverages, medications, cosmetics, professional toxins, and insect bites create allergic reactions on the lips that manifest as swelling, redness, rushes, or ulcers.

Tumors
- A Fibroma is a benign soft tissue that is white, pink, or reddish-blue in color. The most common places to find fibromas are on the top or sides of the tongue, the inside of the cheeks, or anywhere on the lips. Fibromas primarily develop from repeatedly biting the area, an irritation caused by a foreign object, or a trauma to the surrounding tissue. [20]
- Cancer. Lip cancer develops from abnormal cells that grow out of control and form lesions or tumors on the lips. Lip cancer is a type of oral cancer. It develops in thin, flat cells, which are termed squamous cells. Non- melanoma skin cancers are comprised of 95% squamous cell carcinomas and 5% basal cell carcinomas. [21]

2. Diseases of the Lips in Eastern Medicine

Face reading (physiognomy) has been an important component in making a correct diagnosis for over a thousand years in Traditional Chinese Medicine. [22] According to the theory of the Five Elements in TCM, the different parts of the face belong to different organs. The ears, under eye region, philtrum, and chin belong to the Kidney (Water element). The Liver (Wood element) includes the eyebrows, temples, and jaw. The eyes, tip of the tongue, nose, and wrinkles belong to the Heart (Fire element). The mouth, upper lip, and lower cheek belong to the Spleen and Stomach (Earth element). The nose, cheekbones, and skin belong to the Lung (Metal element). [22]

Changes in shape, color, and turgor, as well as the formation of spots or wrinkles on different parts of the face were connected with specific hereditary or acquired pathologic processes and characteristic personal features.

In accordance with human physiognomy, various emotions (endogenic etiology factors in TCM) form wrinkles on parts of the face and form an emotional map that can be read by the practitioner. [22]

In TCM, the lips belong to the Spleen and Stomach element. Lips that are strong, full, tight, moist, and have good turgor indicate a strong spleen and stomach. Thin, dry, and flaccid lips are a sign of spleen deficiency. Very full, dark, overly moist, and puffy lips are indicative of dampness and stagnation that causes the patient to gain weight easily. A large, full, wide mouth is a sign of a healthy appetite and the desire to ingest physical and mental nourishment. This type of formation is more sensual, as well, and signals generosity and the capacity to give to others.

People with small mouths and thinner lips are more introverted and are less openhanded. When the upper lip is larger than the lower lip, a predisposition for emotional irritation exists. When the lower lip is fuller than the upper lip, the person revels in sensual pleasure (delicious food and drink, an attractive home, and a congenial environment). Firm lips are a sign of good muscle tone in the digestive organs, diaphragm, and indicate great self-control and discipline. Poor self-control and lasciviousness is indicated when the lower lip is lax. [22]

The zone that represents stomach function is above the upper lip on either side of the philtrum. When the zone is full, pink, and has good turgor, stomach function is good. When the zone is hollow, with decreased turgor, stomach function is deficient. If the zone is overly tight, the patient is on a restricted calorie diet. The redness of the zone is a sign of excess fire in the stomach (from eating hot and spicy foods). A white zone indicates a frozen stomach (from eating raw foods, ice cream, and consuming ice-cold beverages). If the zone is dark, the patient has stomach stagnation. The formation of multiple vertical lines above the upper lip is a sign of selflessness and caring for others before oneself. Vertical lines below the lower lip indicate a bitter disposition. Vertical wrinkles on the side of the mouth are signs of disappointment. Laughing, smiling, and a sense of humor form vertical lines on the lower lip. [22]

The area between the nose and mouth is called the philtrum. In TCM a wide, long, and deep philtrum indicates fertility and creativity.

SECTION V

MANIFESTATIONS OF PATHOLOGIC PROCESSES OF THE LIPS

When analyzing pathologic changes of the lip organ zones, which are the projections of pathologic processes and diseases in the internal organs and tissues, the practitioner has to pay attention, not only to changes in the organ zones, but also to the shape, color, turgor, destructive and proliferative processes of the lips in their entirety, and the surrounding skin.

1. Changes in Lip Shape

The shape of the lips is genetically and racially determined. Lip shape is generally correlated to specific signs pointing to the character of a person. Bigger and unsymmetrical lips are a sign of an intrepid personality; a slightly bigger, arched mouth with equal sized, moderately protruding lips is a sign of self-confidence and persistence; drooping and tight lips are a sign of shyness or shrewdness; hollow and thin lips are indicative of glibness or resentment; well-formed, puffy lips are signs of kindness, sincerity, openness, and cheerfulness; thin lips are a sign of astuteness, egoism, coldness, sarcasm, or insincerity; puffy and childishly formed lips are signs of trustfulness and frankness; a slightly prominent upper lip over the lower lip is a sign of an intelligent, conscientious, and open character. [23]

In TCM, the upper lip belongs to the Spleen element. The zone that represents the stomach function is above the upper lip on either side of the philtrum. [22] Changes in the shape, color, and turgor of these areas give information about the functional activity of the stomach and eating habits of the person. (See IV. 2)

2. Changes in Lip Color

Normal color of the lips is pink to slightly reddish, with a homogenous distribution of color on the upper and lower lips. Changes in the homogenous distribution of color in the reflection zones pertaining to the internal organs is indicative of the manifestation of an inadequate perfusion of blood in the corresponding internal organs. (See Fig. 6)

Fig. 6 Normal Lip Color

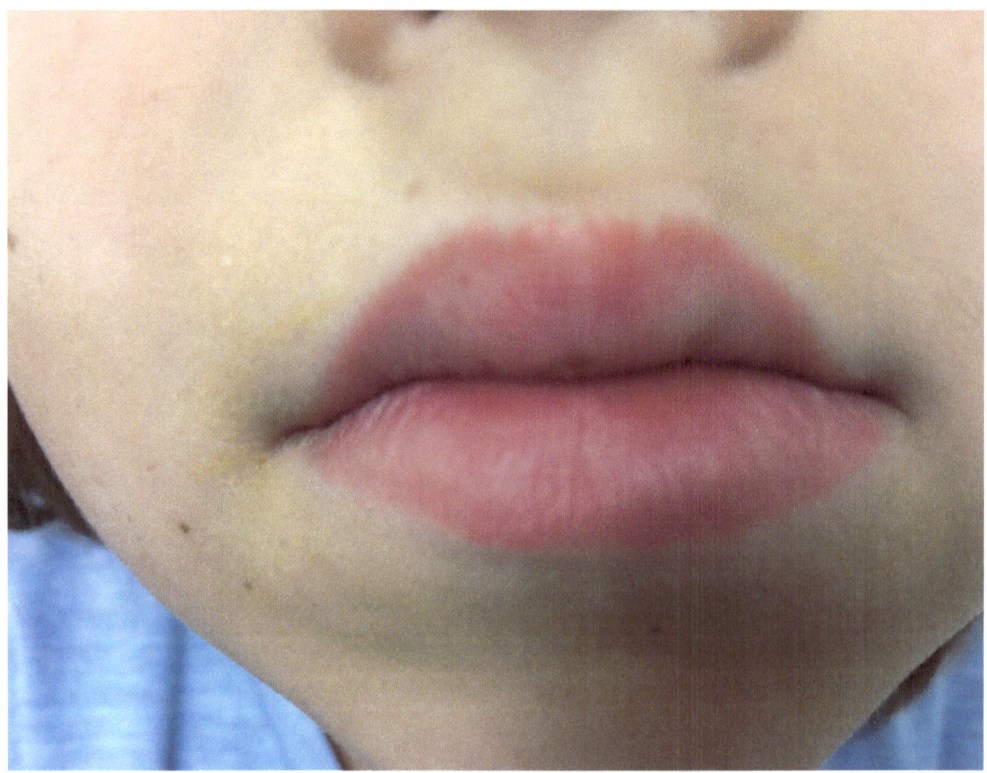

Red and dark red spots represent acute infection, inflammation, and overuse of stimulants. Red spots (located in the reflection zones pertaining to the internal organs) or redness of the upper and lower lips (indicating the entire body) with swelling are symptoms of an allergic reaction in the corresponding regions. (See Fig. 7)

Fig. 7 Red Lip Color

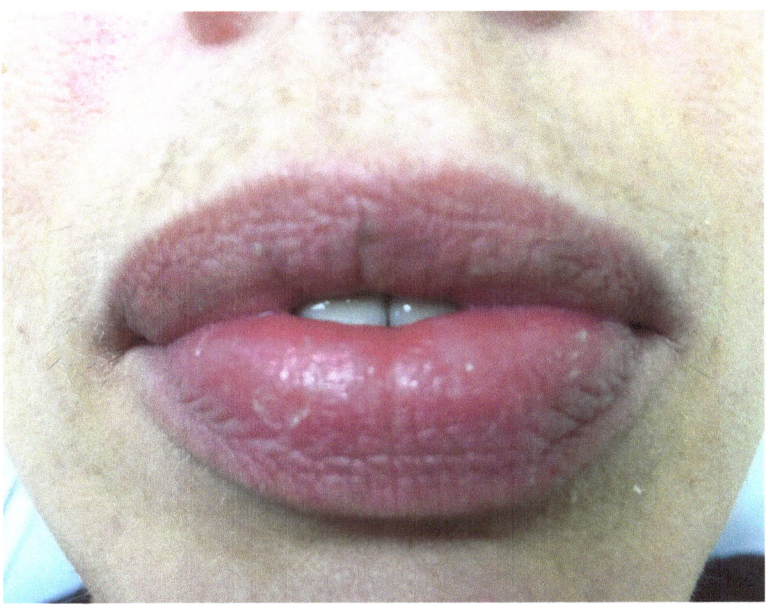

Blue spots (located in the reflection zones pertaining to the internal organs) or a blue-purplish lip color (indicative of the entire body) demonstrates the manifestation of blood stasis in the corresponding regions. (See Fig. 8 a, b)

Fig. 8a Blue Lip Color and Blue Spots

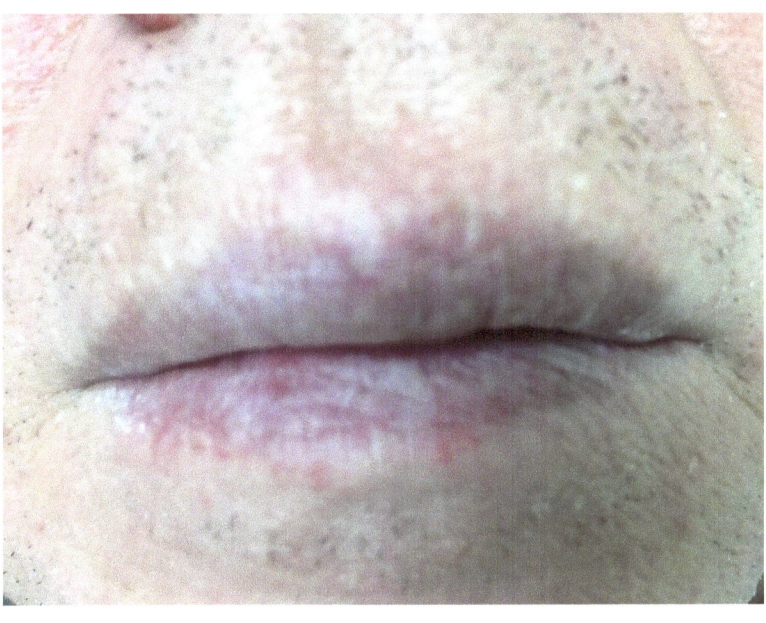

Fig 8b

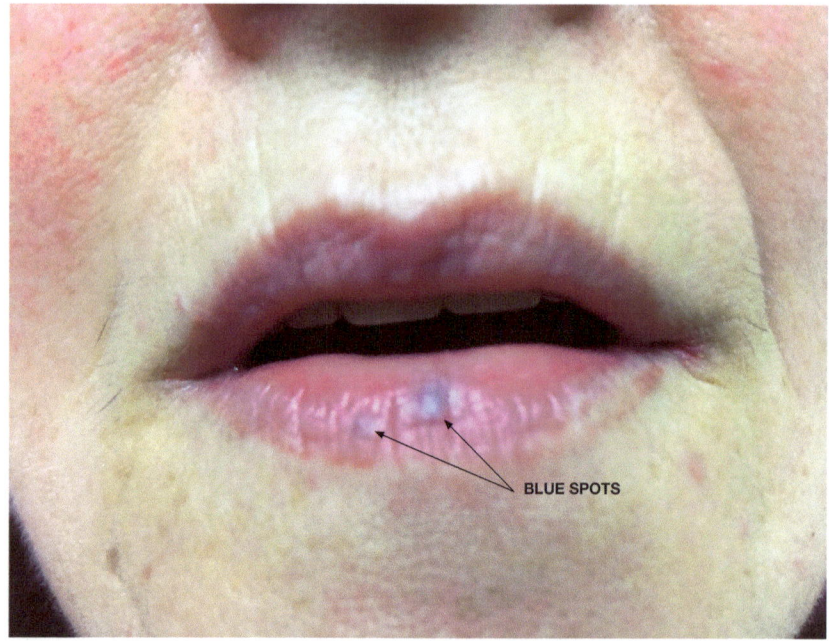

A light pink lip is a characteristic sign of anemia. (See Fig. 9)

Fig. 9 Light pink lip color

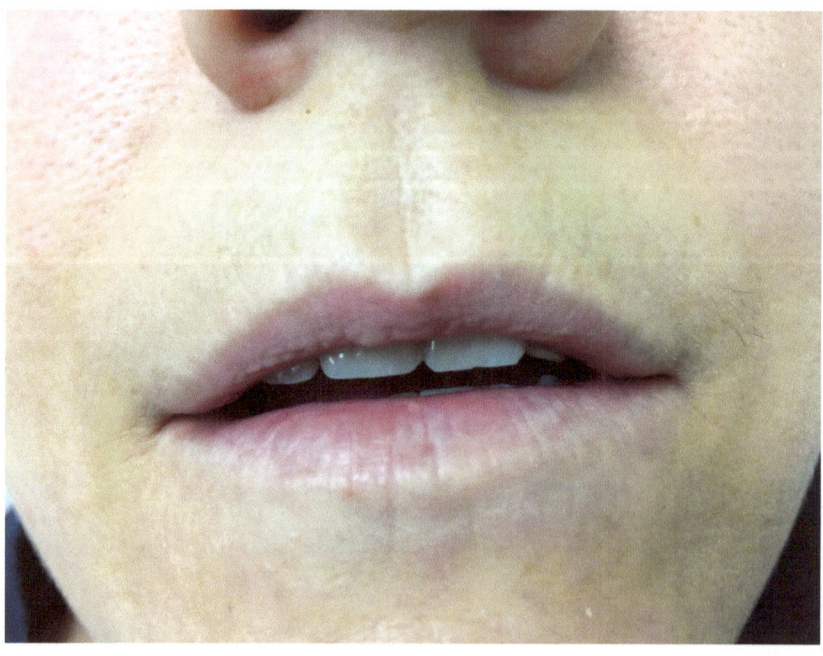

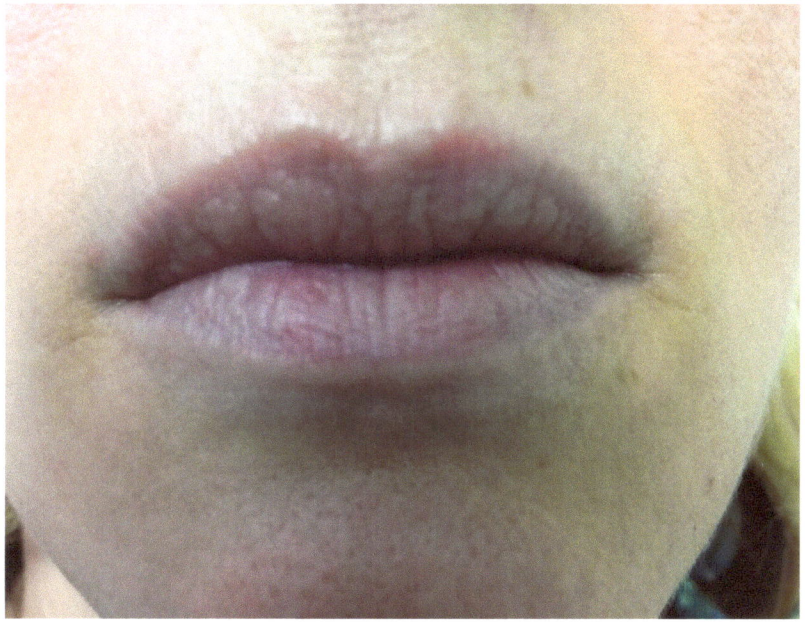

Brown and black spots are formed after a pathologic process of long duration that resulted in significant structural changes, such as fractures, cysts, tumors, and the replacement of functional tissue with connective tissue. (See Fig. 10)

Fig. 10a Brown Spot on the Lips

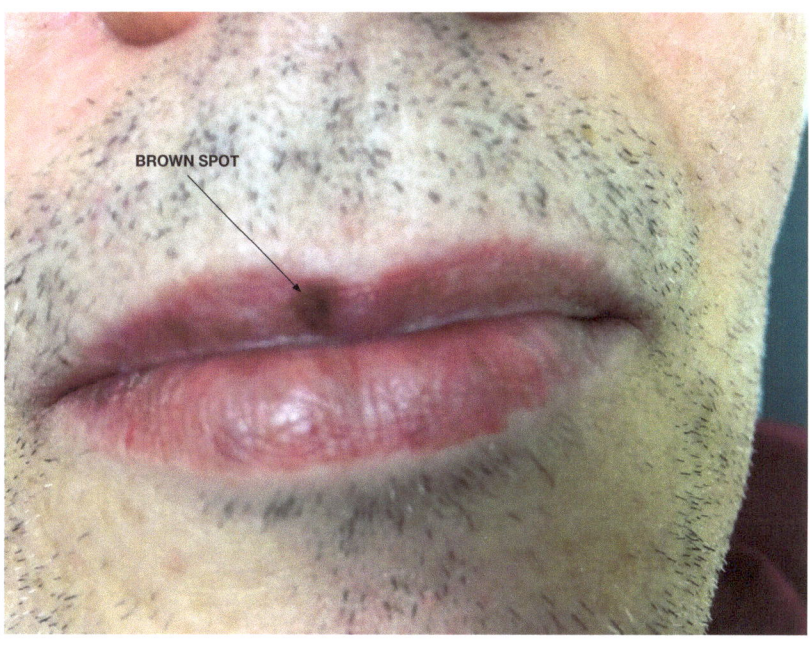

Lip Diagnostics

Fig 10b Black Spot on the Lips

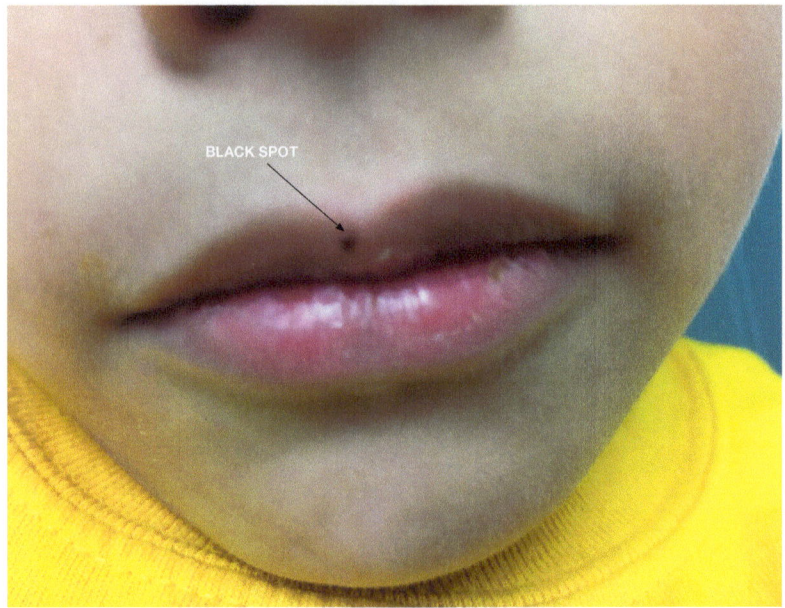

White spots and lines on the lip reflection zones represent decreased functional activity of the corresponding internal organs (See Fig. 11).

Fig. 11 White Spot on the Lips

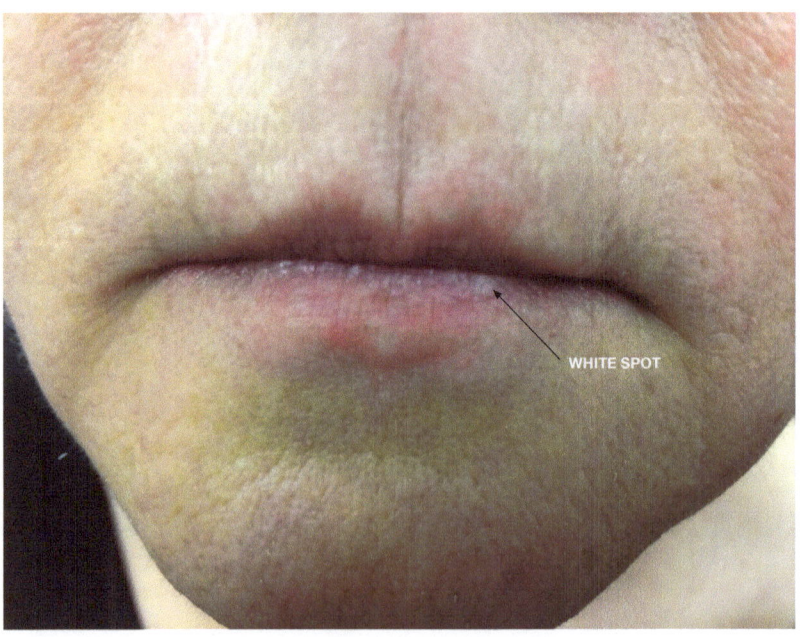

24   *Manifestations of Pathologic Processes of the Lips*

3. Changes in Turgor

Decreased turgor of the lips can be seen due to dehydration, malnutrition, or decreased blood perfusion. Increased turgor is a sign of infection, allergy, stimulants, fluid retention, or hypertension.

Fig. 12 Increased Turgor of the Lips

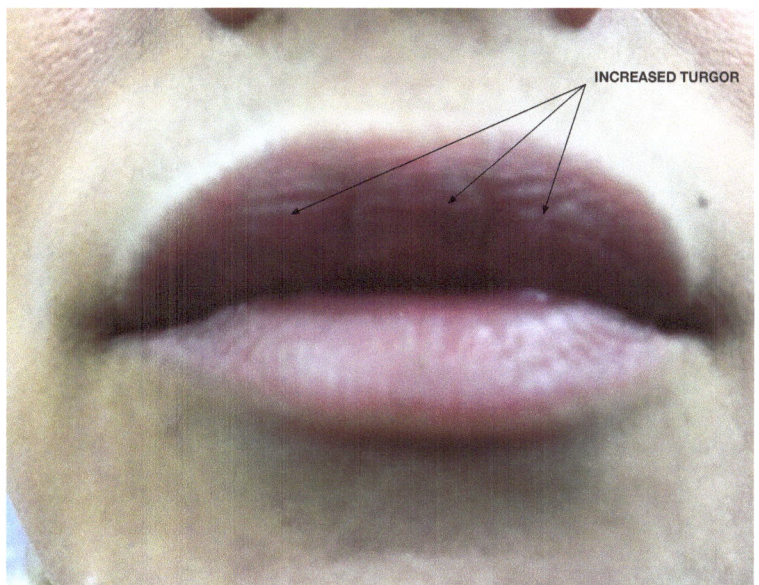

Fig. 13 Decreased Lip Turgor

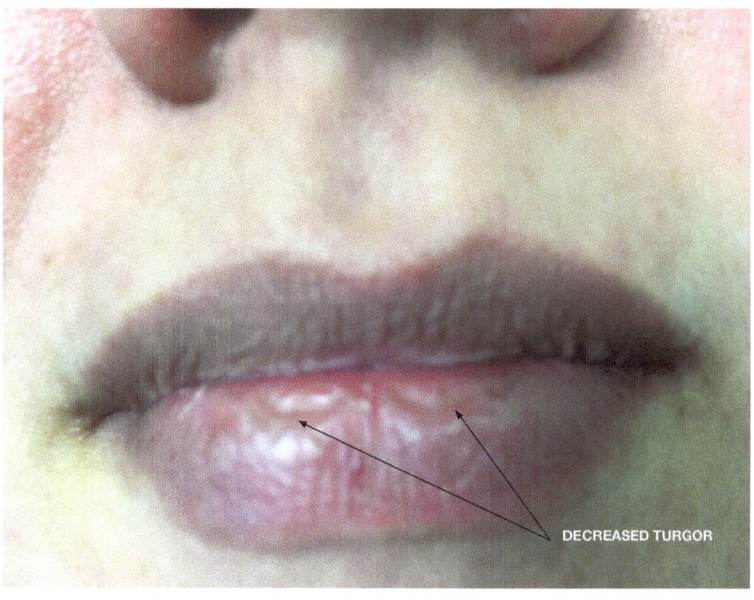

4. Destructive and Proliferative Processes

Destructive changes on the lip reflection zones pertaining to the internal organs are manifestations of existing, or old, pathologic processes which led to the replacement of the normal structure of corresponding organs with connective tissue. This process occurs after infections, intoxication, nutritional deficits, and surgical procedures. Such changes in the lip reflection zones appear as folds, cracks, or scars (See Fig. 14).

Fig. 14 Folds and Cracks on the Lips

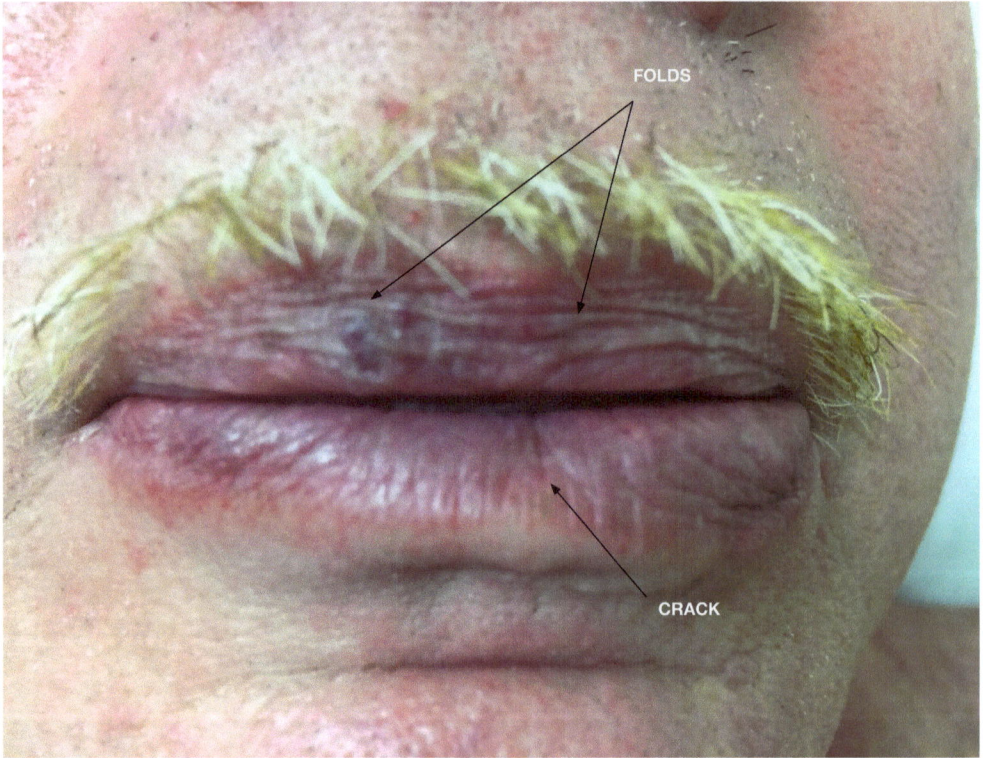

Proliferative processes on the lips can be the result of local process such as fibromas, squamous cell, and basal cell carcinomas, or can be the manifestation of proliferative processes within the internal organs that are reflected on the lip zones. The proliferative processes of the internal organs (cysts, polyps, fibromas, tumors, and stones) are present as very small bumps in the lip reflection zones. (See Fig. 15)

Fig. 15a Bumps on the Lips

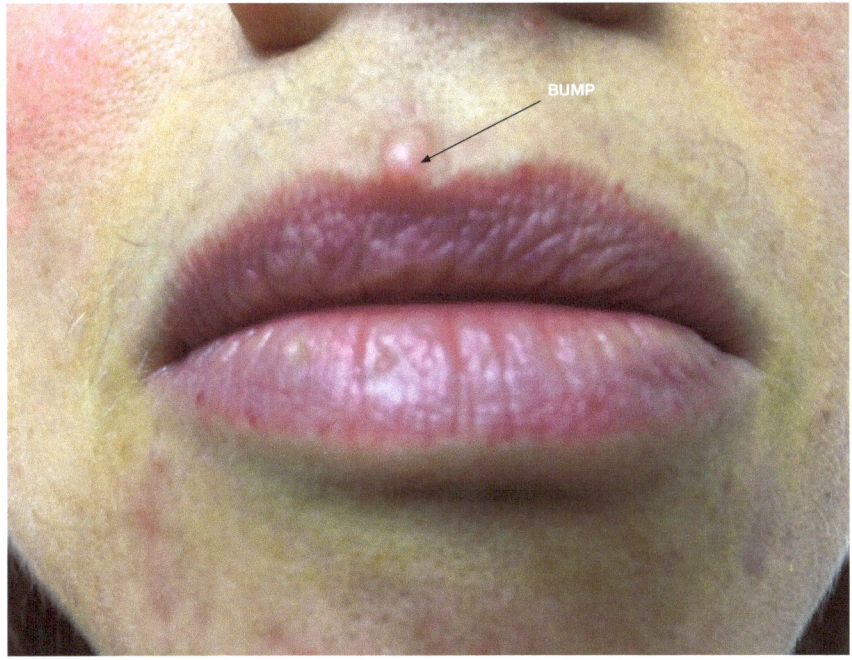

Fig. 15b Bumps on the Lips

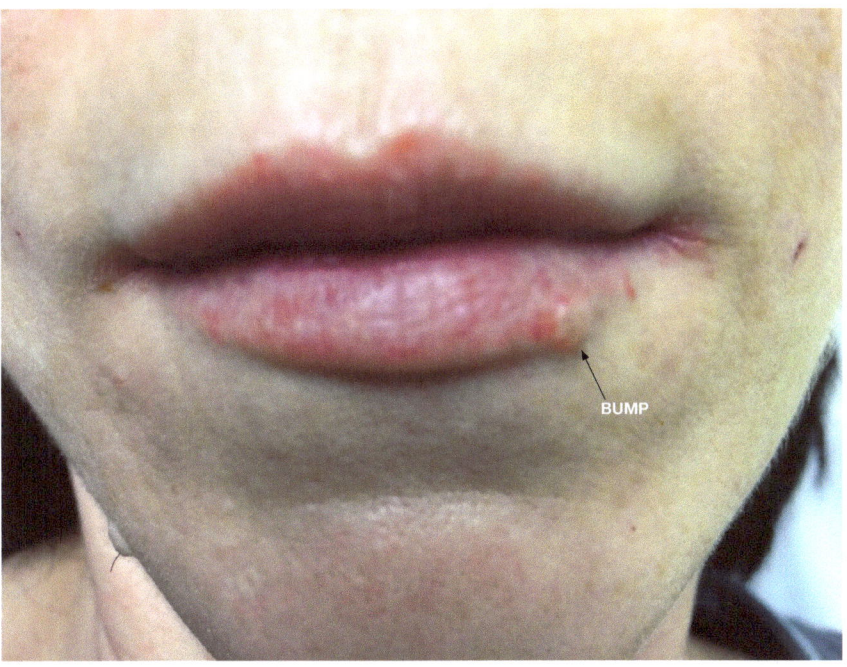

5. Changes in the Skin Around the Lips

When a pathologic process leaves significant changes in the internal organs and a long period of time had passed (five, ten, fifteen or more years), the spot formed on the lip reflection zone can "travel" to the skin around the lip. The older the pathologic process forming the spot, the further the movement away from the organ reflection zone on the lips. At the same time, a thin line or crack connecting the reflection organ zone on the lip and the spot on the skin can be seen. (See Fig. 16, 17, 18)

Fig. 16 represents a patient with severe trauma to the right knee, which occurred twenty-seven years ago. Note the darker line on the right knee reflection zone and the yellowish bump, which has been travelling from the knee reflection zone to below the lower lip for twenty-seven years.

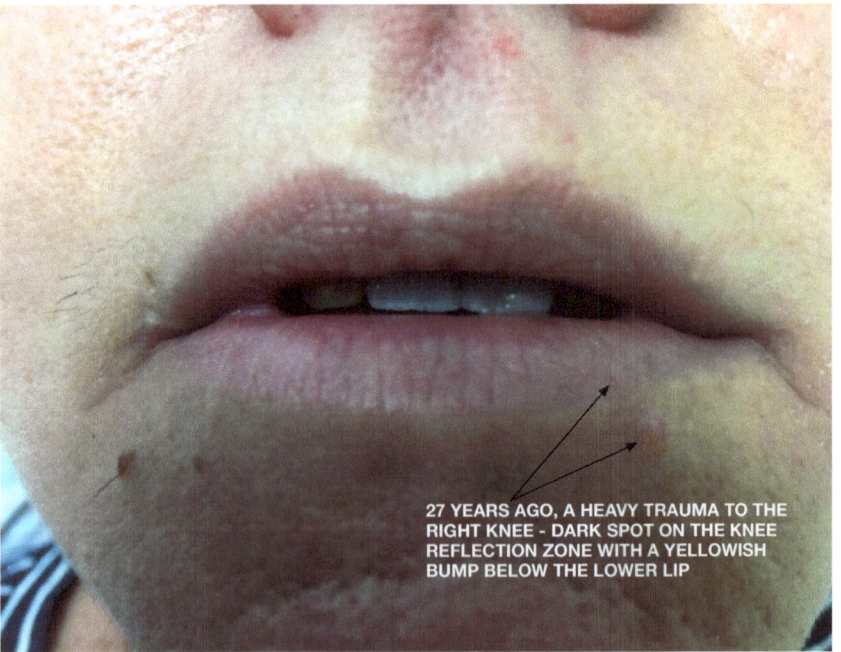

Fig. 17 Small Red Bump Above the Upper Lip. Ten years ago the patient had surgery on the right lung for cancer and chronic pleuritis. The bump moved from the right lung reflection zone to above the lip.

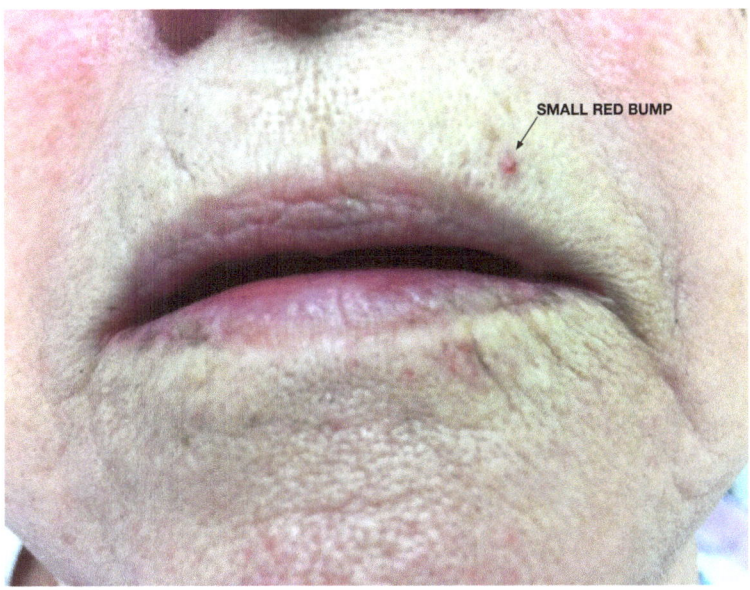

Fig. 18 Some bumps around the lips are signs of predisposition to genetic diseases or the manifestation of the parents' diseases. There are persons who are born with bumps. The patient below was born with a bump above the upper lip. Her mother had hypertonia and a stroke right before she was born.

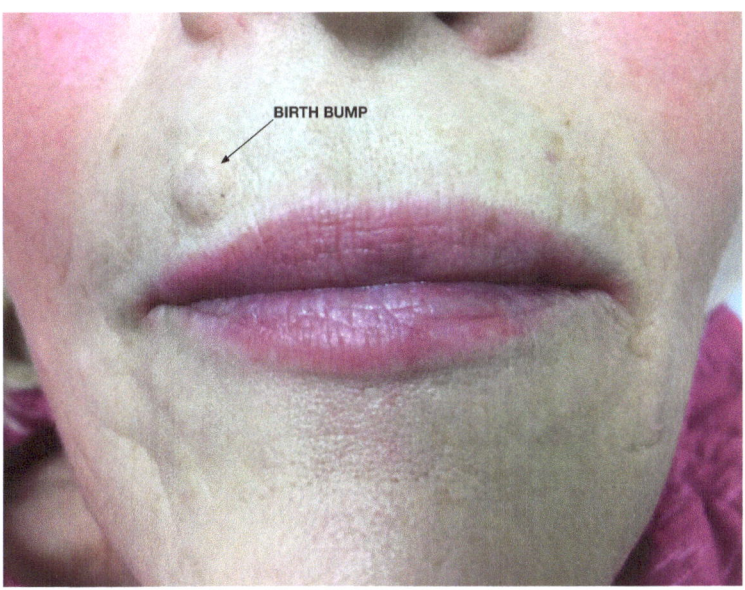

SECTION VI
MANIFESTATIONS OF THE DISEASES ON THE LIP ORGAN ZONES

1. Pathologic Processes of the Pulmonary System

1.1. Infections of the Upper Respiratory System – Nose, Sinuses, Pharynx

Fig. 19 The photo below is of a patient with frequent infections of the nose, sinuses, tonsils, and pharynx. Currently, he is suffering from a bacterial infection of the upper respiratory system that is spreading to the eyes and is causing severe headaches. Note the mosaic pattern of red and light pink to white spots on the reflection zones corresponding to the nose, throat, eyes, and brain.

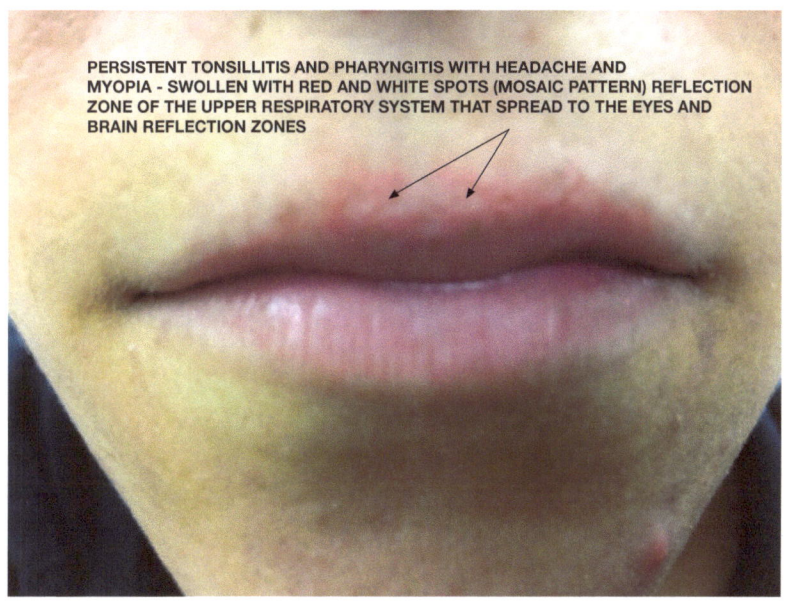

Fig. 20 The image below is of a patient with an acute viral infection of the nose, sinuses, throat, and bronchi, which induces severe neck and shoulder pain. Note the red spots on the reflection zones corresponding to the upper respiratory system, neck, and shoulders.

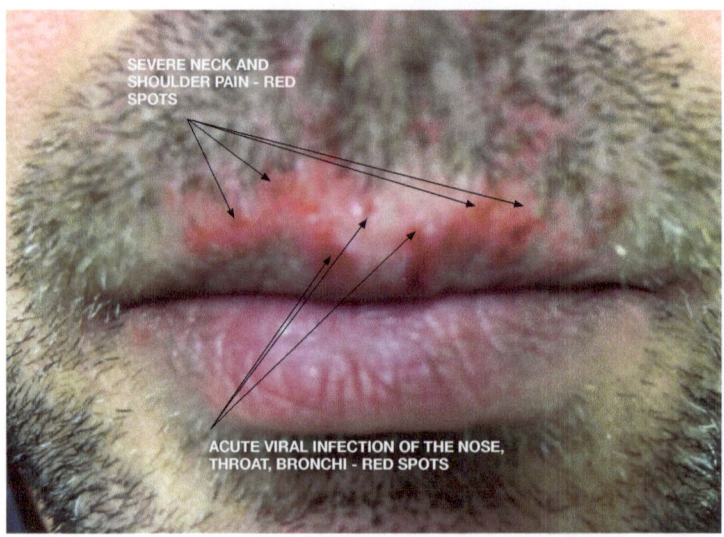

Fig. 21 The patient below has had chronic tonsillitis since childhood. The patient was on antibiotics when the photograph was taken. Chronic infections of the upper respiratory system induced replacement of the normal lip membrane with white colored skin. Note the swollen, red, and yellowish spots on the right tonsil reflection zone.

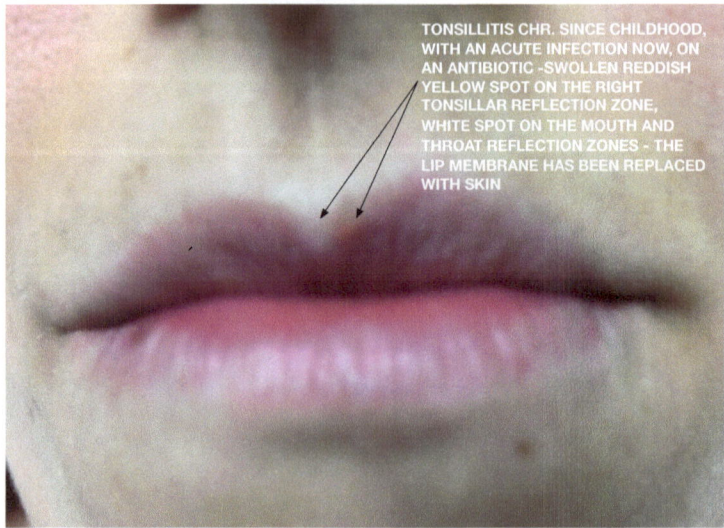

Fig.22 a. The patient below had multiple episodes of tonsillitis as a child. The normal lip membrane has been replaced with skin within the mouth reflection zone.

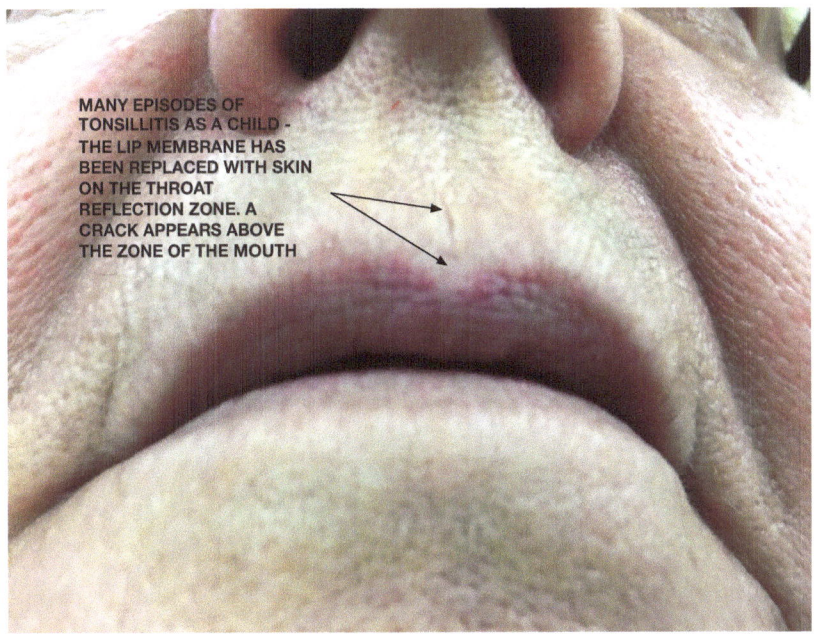

Fig. 22 b

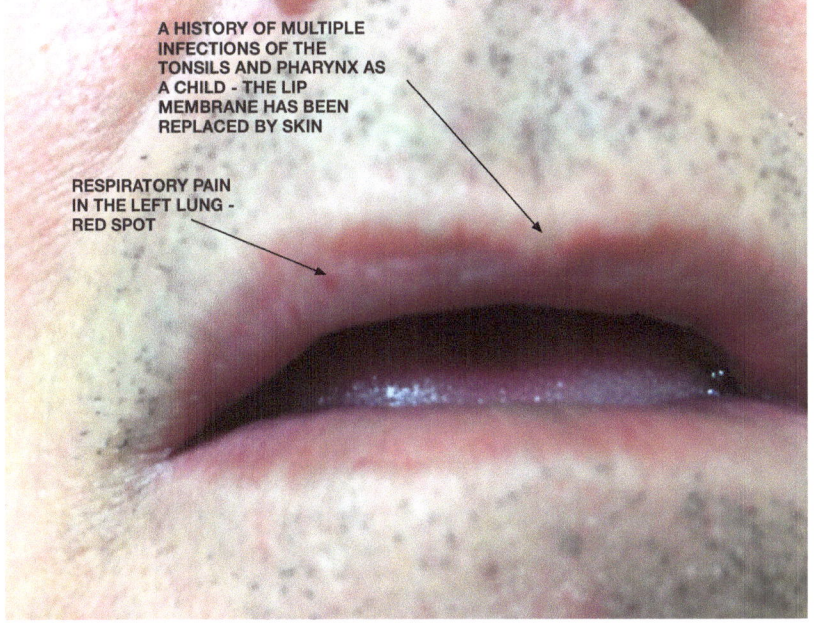

Lip Diagnostics

Fig. 23 Thirty years ago this patient experienced severe tonsillitis that was accompanied by a tonsillectomy, which left a brown spot above the upper lip.

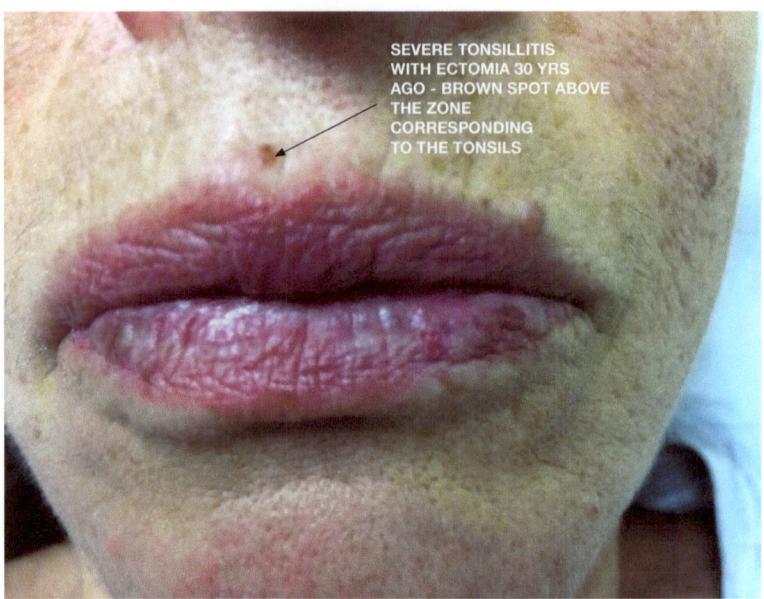

1.2. Infections of the Lower Respiratory System – Bronchus, Lung

Fig. 24 A patient with chronic bronchitis, pictured below, has transversal folds and a swollen purplish spot on the reflection zone corresponding to the left lung.

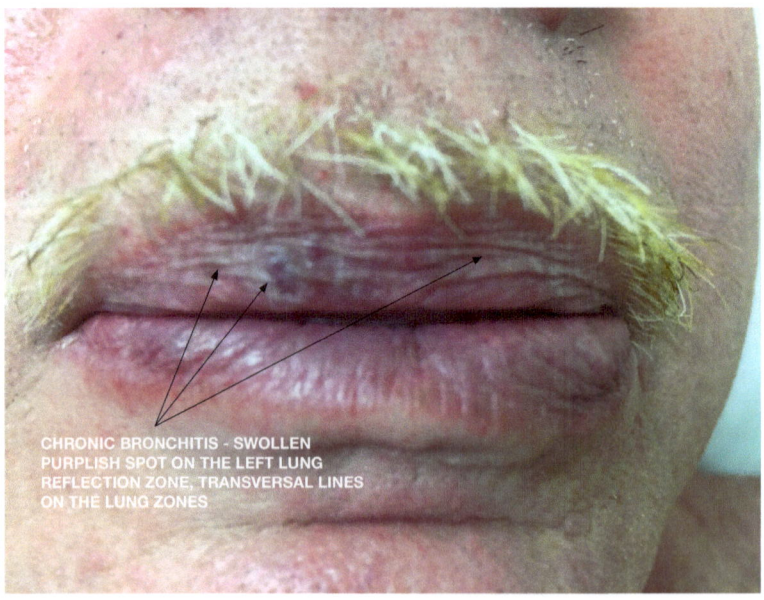

Fig. 25 The patient pictured below experienced pleurisy of the left lung three years ago. Note the red spot on the left pleural reflection zone.

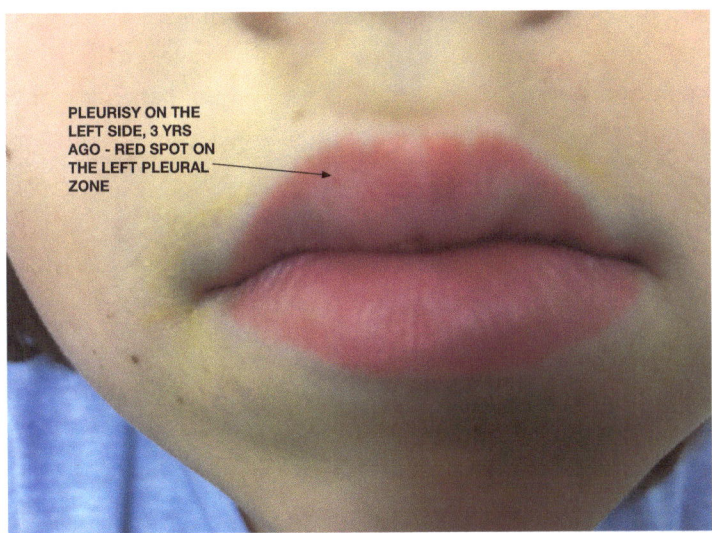

1.3. Allergy Affecting the Upper Respiratory System – Nose, Sinuses, Pharynx

Fig. 26 The patient pictured below has allergic rhino -sinusitis. Note the swollen, darker pink bumps and the line in the nose and sinus reflection zones. The allergic process spread to the eye reflection zones on the left side more than on the right side. Note the darker pink bump on the left eye reflection zone.

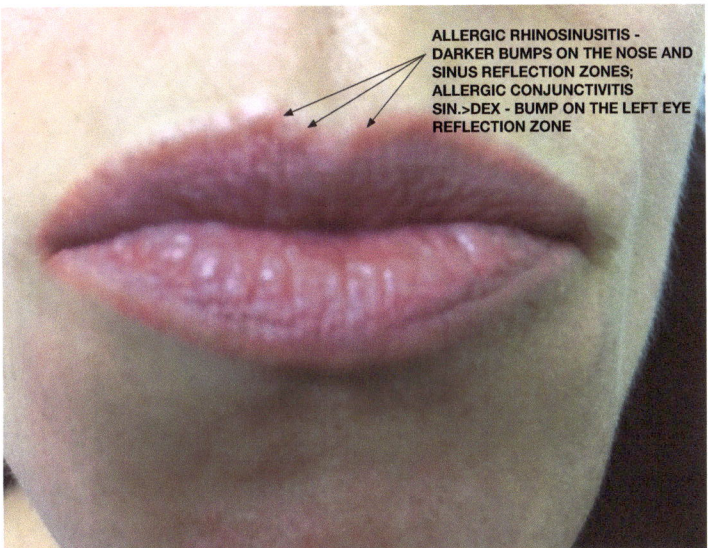

Fig. 27 The patient below experienced an allergic process in the upper respiratory system within the first year of life. Later the allergic processes spread to the lungs and the patient developed asthma. This child was born with a black spot within the reflection zone corresponding to the upper respiratory system. Eating sweet foods depressed the immune system. Note the red spot on the pancreatic reflection zone.

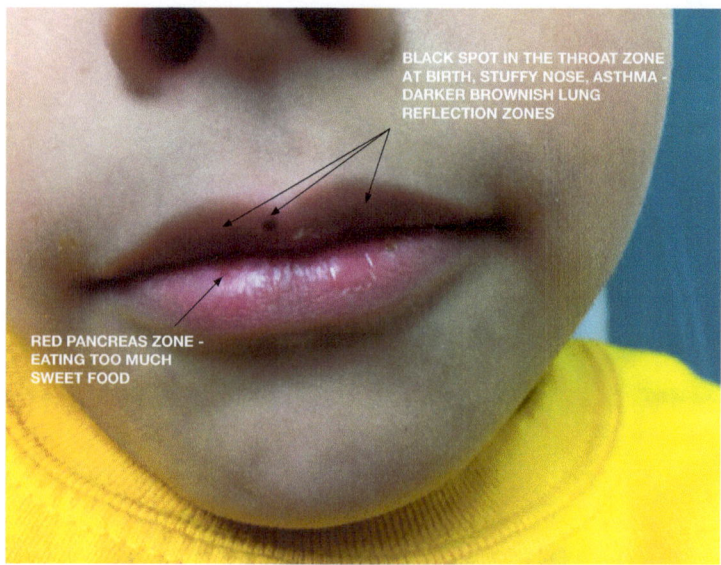

Fig. 28 The patient below has a seasonal allergy, and rhinosinusitis. Note the reddish-pink nasal, sinus, and throat reflection zones. The swollen, purplish spleen reflection zone is a manifestation of an overactive immune system.

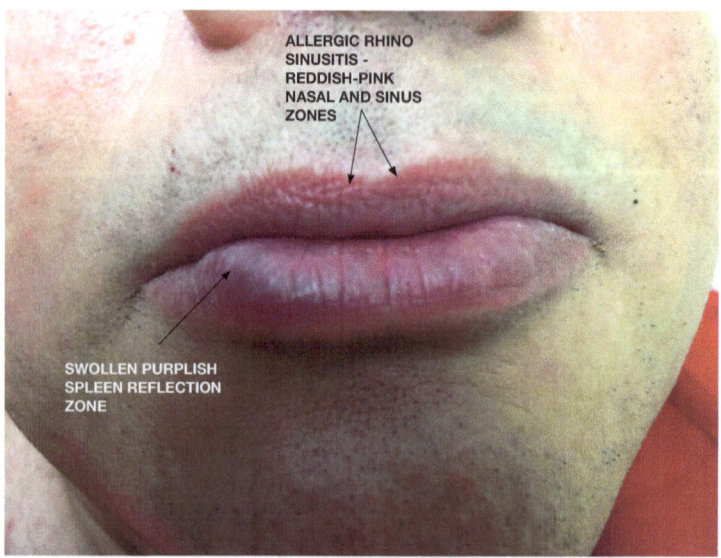

1.4. Allergy of the Lower Respiratory System – bronchus, lung

Fig. 29 The patient below has a thirty-five year history of asthma. Note the many yellowish spots and bumps in the nose, throat, and lung reflection zones. His splenomegaly can be seen within the reddish, slightly swollen spleen reflection zone.

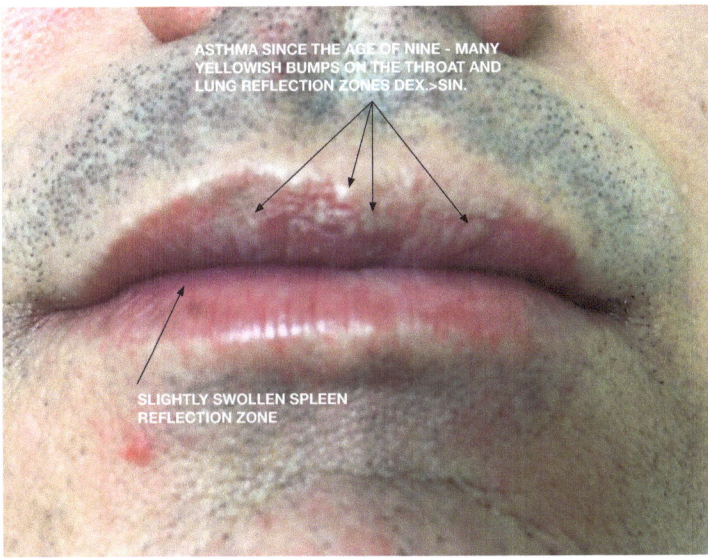

Fig. 30 The patient below has chronic allergic bronchitis, indicated by the light yellowish lung reflection zones. The right lung reflection zone is larger than the left lung zone and contains more spots, which are light brown in color.

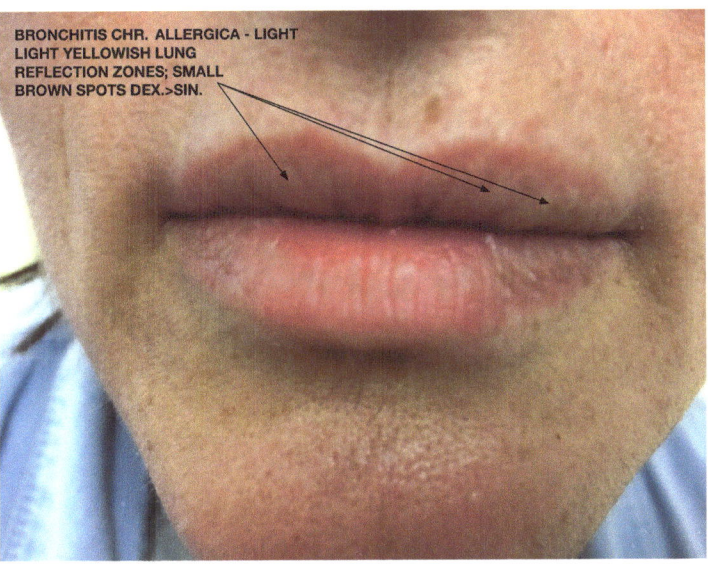

Fig.31 The patient below experienced asthma during childhood. The asthmatic condition was treated but left a prominent brown spot on the left bronchial reflection zone. Light brown spots can be seen on the lung reflection zones. There are more of them on the left than on the right side.

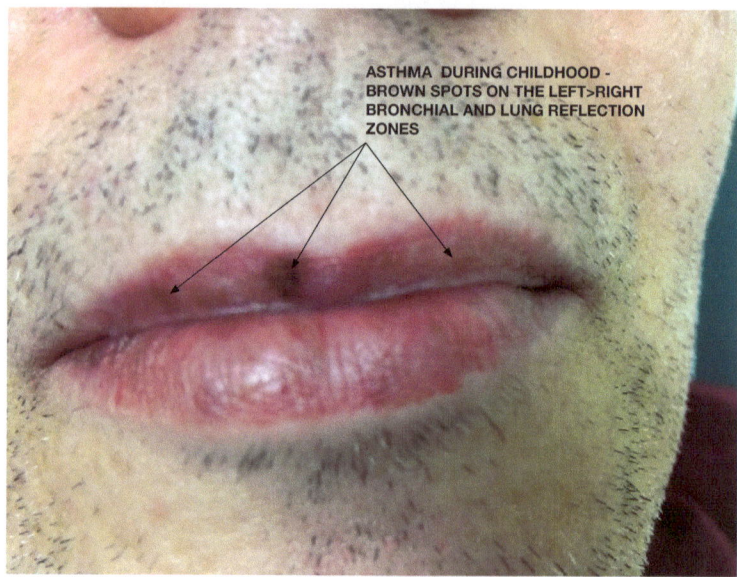

Fig. 32 The patient below has chronic bronchitis, a persistent cough, and pain in the right lung. The lung reflection zones contain white spots, and the right side is bigger than the left side.

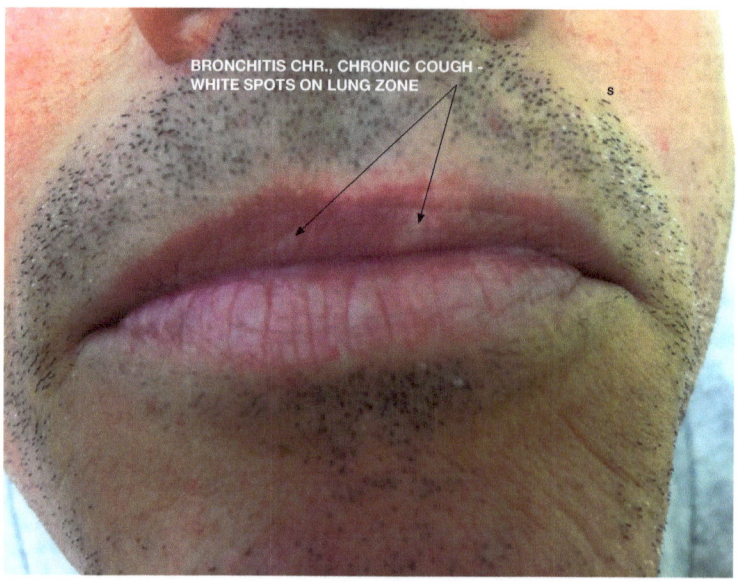

1.5. Proliferative Process of the Lung – Replacing Functional Tissue with Connective tissue; Tumors

Fig. 33 .1.2 The patient below was diagnosed with pneumosclerosis ten years ago. Multiple 5-6 mm nodules stemming from an autoimmune reaction to inhaled toxins (construction materials) were discovered in the lungs. Note the numerous yellowish bumps within the lung reflection zones. The patient is suffering from hepatosplenomegaly indicated by the slightly swollen, purplish liver and spleen reflection zones. There is a black spot on the liver reflection zone. See Fig.33.2

Fig. 33.1

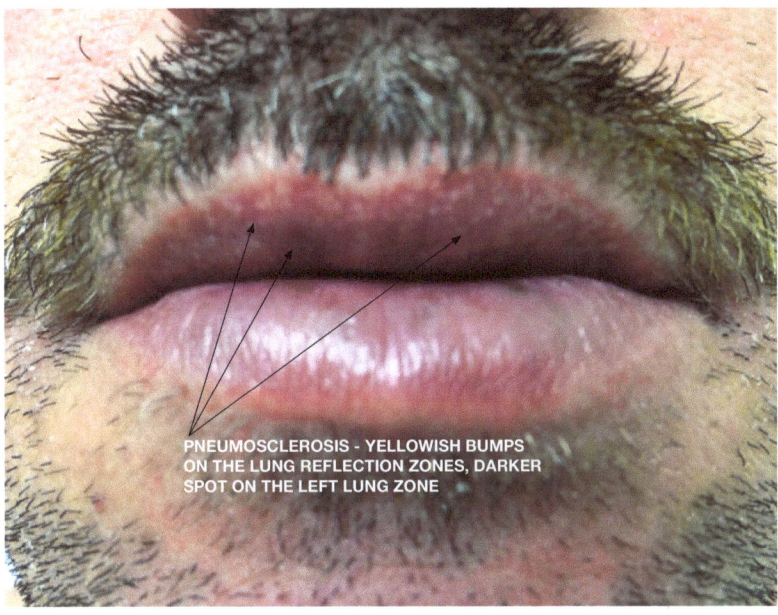

Fig. 33.2

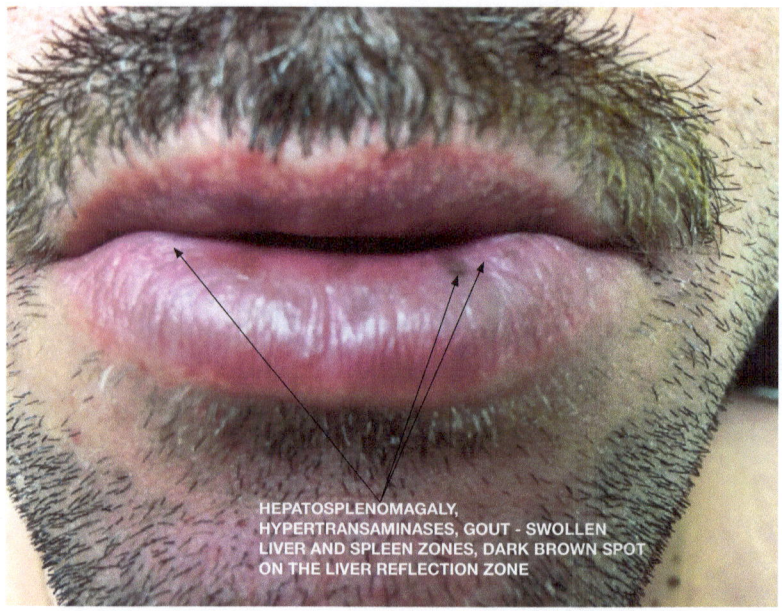

HEPATOSPLENOMAGALY, HYPERTRANSAMINASES, GOUT - SWOLLEN LIVER AND SPLEEN ZONES, DARK BROWN SPOT ON THE LIVER REFLECTION ZONE

Fig. 34 The patient below was diagnosed with cancer of the left breast that metastasized to the left and right lungs. Note the purplish areas with transversal lines on the lung reflection zones and the light red point on the left breast reflection zone.

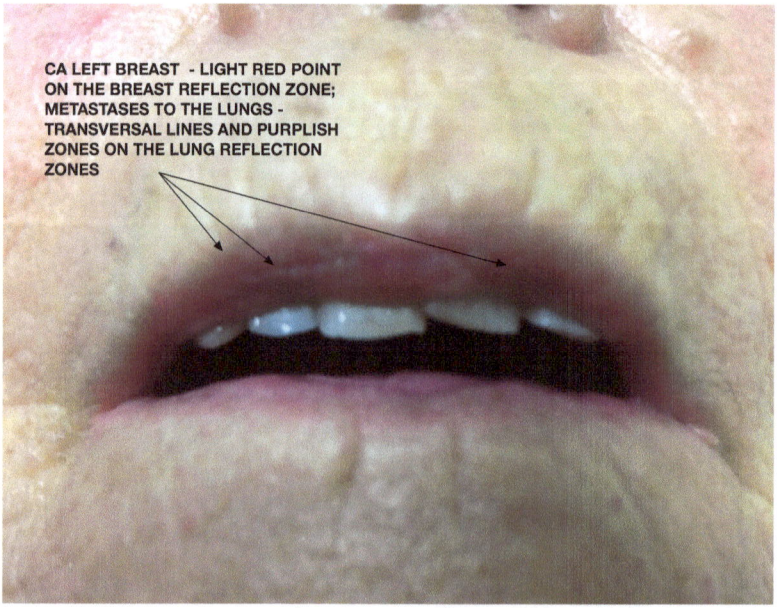

CA LEFT BREAST - LIGHT RED POINT ON THE BREAST REFLECTION ZONE; METASTASES TO THE LUNGS - TRANSVERSAL LINES AND PURPLISH ZONES ON THE LUNG REFLECTION ZONES

Fig. 35 The patient below has pleurisy and cancer of the right lung. The cancerous process is reflected as a small white point on the light whitish- purple right lung reflection zone. The pneumosclerotic process is manifested as a transversal line on the right and left lung reflection zones. The pleurisy is seen in the small red line on the peripheral part of the lung zone. Note the red bump above the upper lip, which formed at the same time as the pleurisy and moved upward from the lung border line over time.

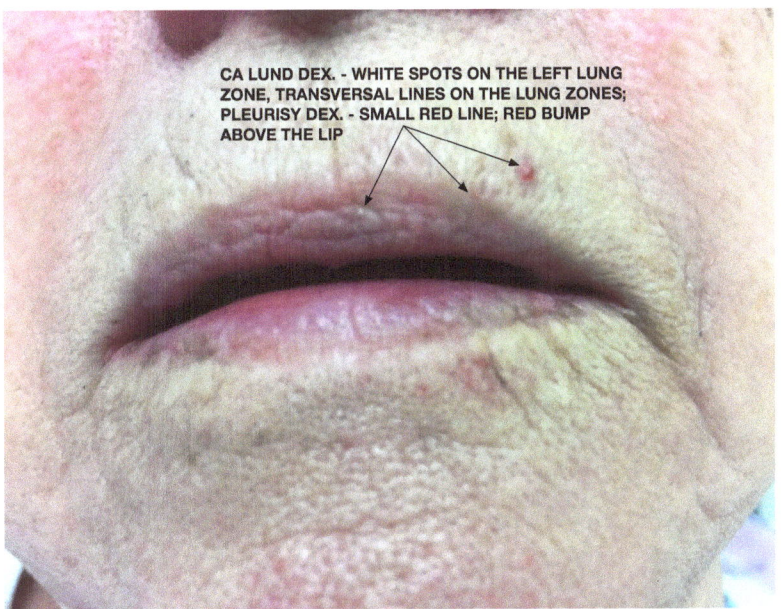

1.6. Influence of Toxins on the Lungs

Photos of the lips of patients who were exposed to various toxins are presented in Section 1.6.

Inhaling a variety of toxins creates changes in the color and turgor of the lips and causes the formation of transversal lines and bumps in, or shrinkage of, the lung reflection zones. The formation of bumps is a sign of an active proliferative process in the lungs (as a nodule or cyst). Transversal lines are a sign of destruction of the lung tissue. Changes in the color of the lung reflection zones depend on the kinds of toxins that were inhaled.

Fig. 36 The patient below was exposed to petroleum products (benzene, oils) for many decades at work. He has a chronic cough and was diagnosed with chronic bronchitis. A purplish black bump can be seen on the left lung reflection zone and a red crack is present on the right lung reflection zone.

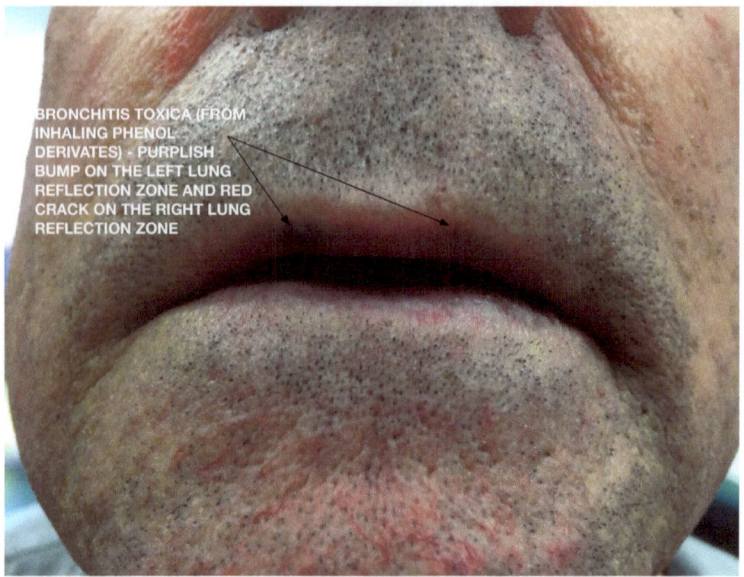

Fig. 37 The patient pictured below exhibited toxic bronchitis after inhaling paint fumes while doing construction work. The lung reflection zone is whitish-gray in color and contains multiple small white bumps.

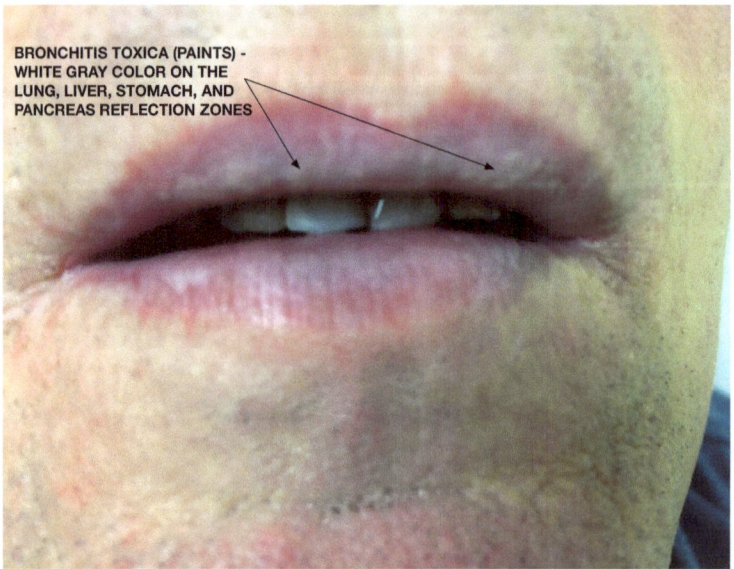

Fig. 38 The patient below developed bronchitis toxicity after inhaling varnishes and paint fumes. The lung reflection zones are of a purplish color and contain dark spots.

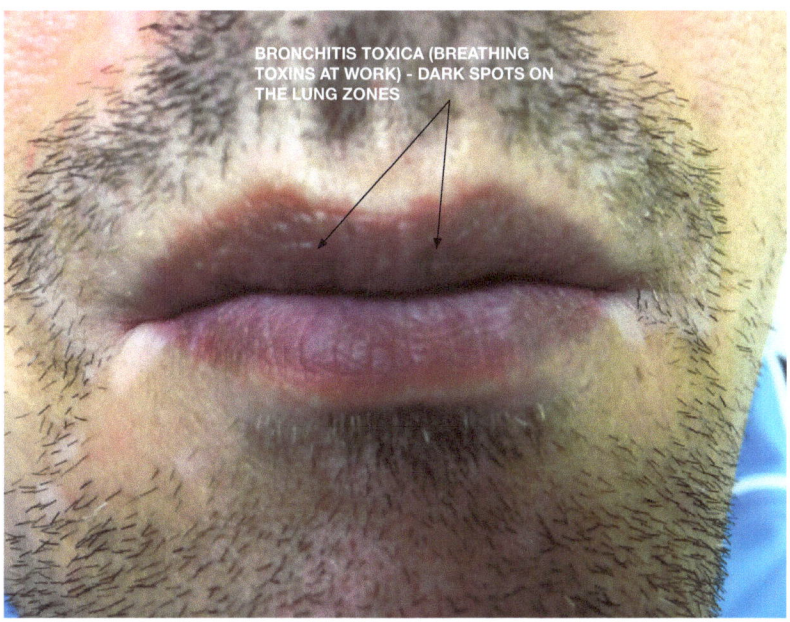

Fig. 40 The patient below developed toxic bronchitis while working in a chemical laboratory. Transversal lines, shrinkage of the lung reflection zones, and white colored lung zones can be seen on the lips.

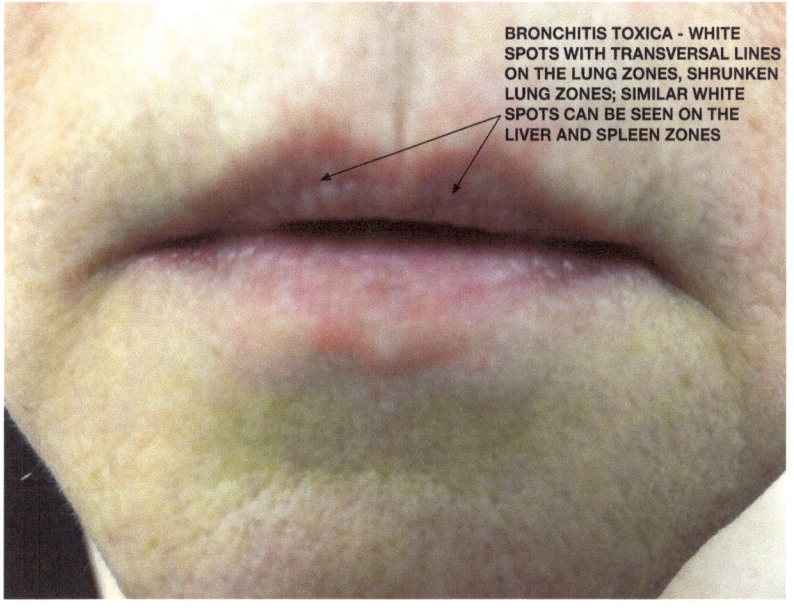

Lip Diagnostics

Fig. 41 The patient below has light yellowish bumps on the lung reflection zones that developed after exposure to various toxins during a war.

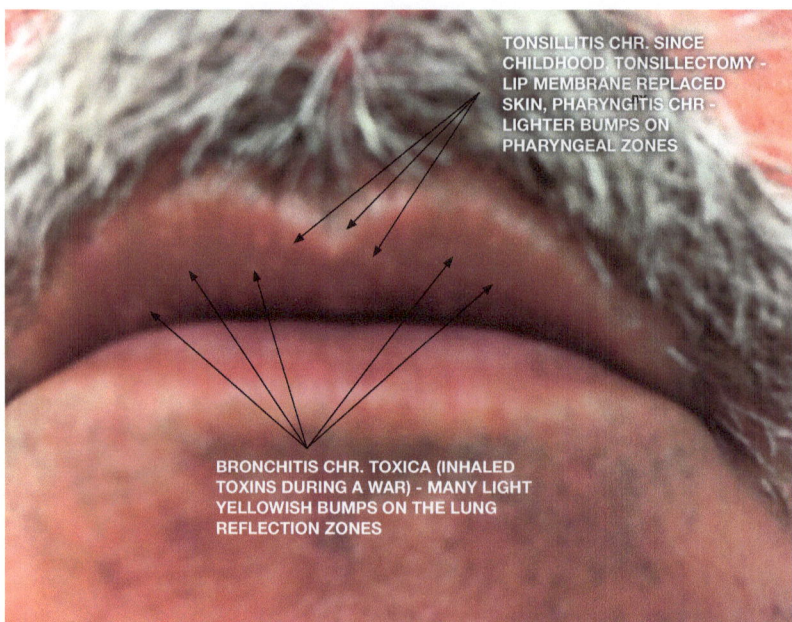

Fig. 42 The lungs of this patient were exposed to oil paint toxins. The lung reflection zones are dark gray in color and contain transversal lines.

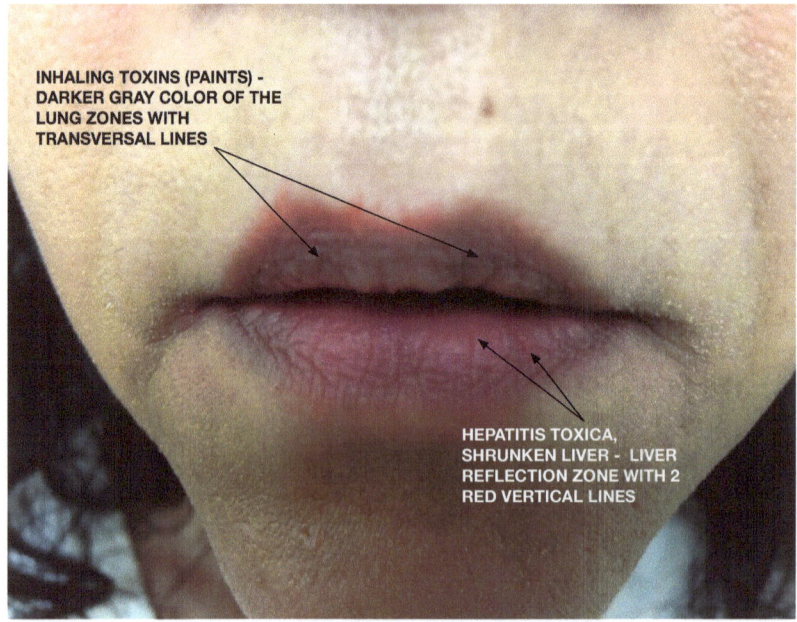

1.7 Sports Activity

Fig. 43 This patient's lung reflection zones (marked by the black points) became enlarged after very intensive and regular sports activity.

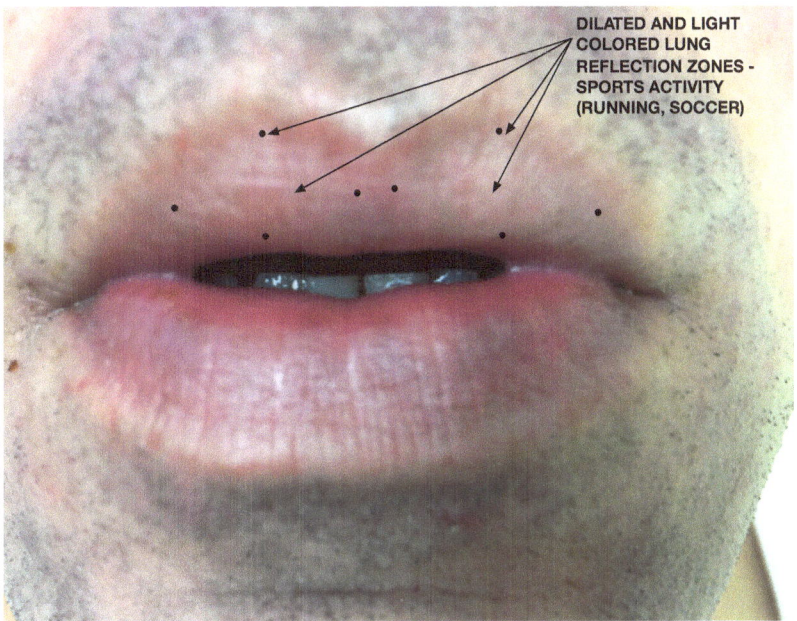

2. Pathologic Processes of the Cardiovascular System

2.1. Hypertension

Essential and symptomatic hypertension changes the size of the heart and alters it spatially in cases of hypertrophy of the left camera. Here, hypertension is represented by dilation and swelling of the heart refection zone. The zone is reddish pink in color. When a patient experiences arrhythmia, a line is formed at an angle across the atrial reflection zone.

Lip Diagnostics

Fig. 44 The patient below has been diagnosed with essential hypertension and supraventricular arrhythmia. The heart reflection zone is red, dilated (marked by the black points), and is swollen. A line forming at an angle in the atrial reflection zone is indicative of arrhythmia (longer arrow). The patient has elevated blood sugar levels, which are represented by the vertical white line on the pancreatic reflection zone.

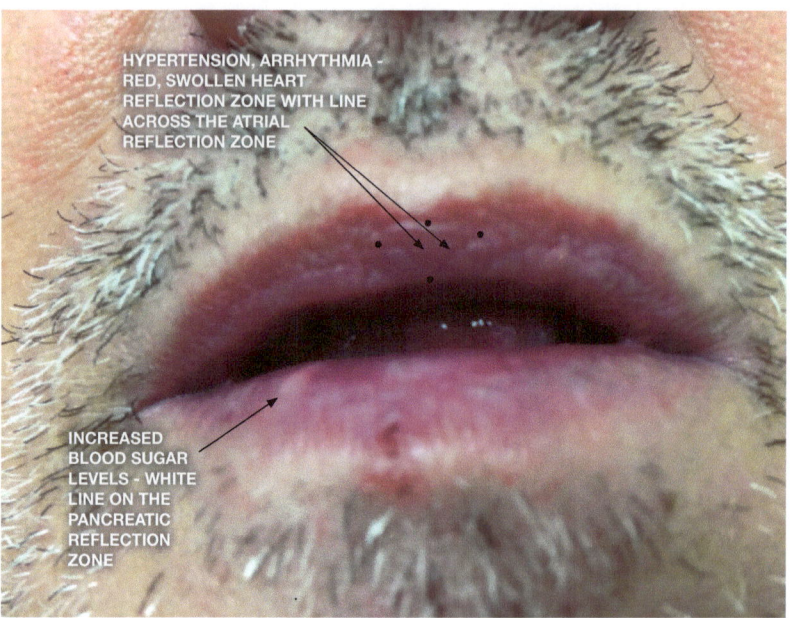

Fig. 45 The patient in the photo below has essential hypertension, arrhythmia, mitral valve prolapse, dyslipidemia, and toxic bronchitis. All the pathologic processes are present - the dilated heart reflection zone (marked by the black dots); the very light angular line on the atrial reflection zone, which is indicative of arrhythmia (longer arrow); the red spot that signals a mitral valve prolapse (shorter arrow). The toxic influence on the lung and heart is indicated by the purplish spots on the left lung and heart reflection zones. The light pinkish yellow spots on the liver reflection zone demonstrate liver steatosis, and dyslipidemia.

New Reflection Zones of the Human Organs on the Lips

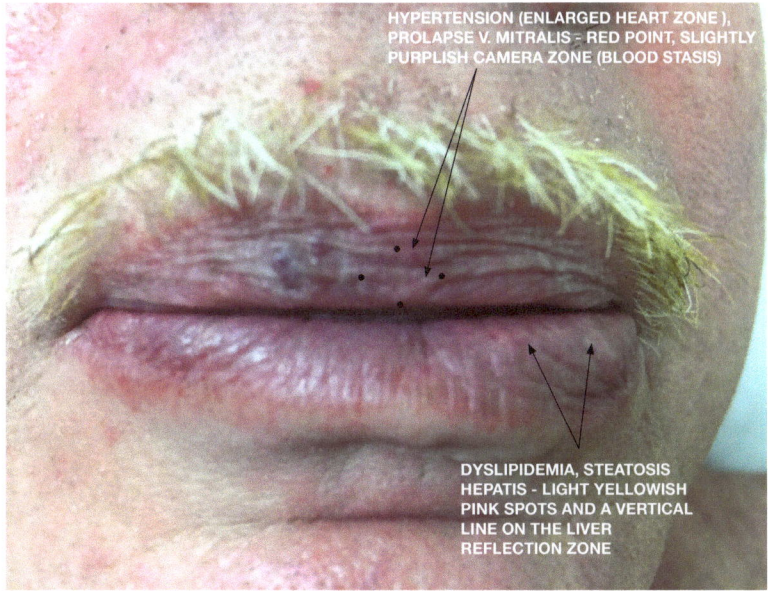

Fig. 46 The patient below has symptomatic hormonal hypertension, and arrhythmia. The heart reflection zone is dilated (marked by the black points), and the darker line seen on the atrial reflection zone is indicative of arrhythmia. The reflection zone corresponding to the right thyroid gland has a tiny hole that is connected by a transversal line to the heart reflection zone. Changes in the hormonal activity of the thyroid gland provoked the irregular rhythm of the heart.

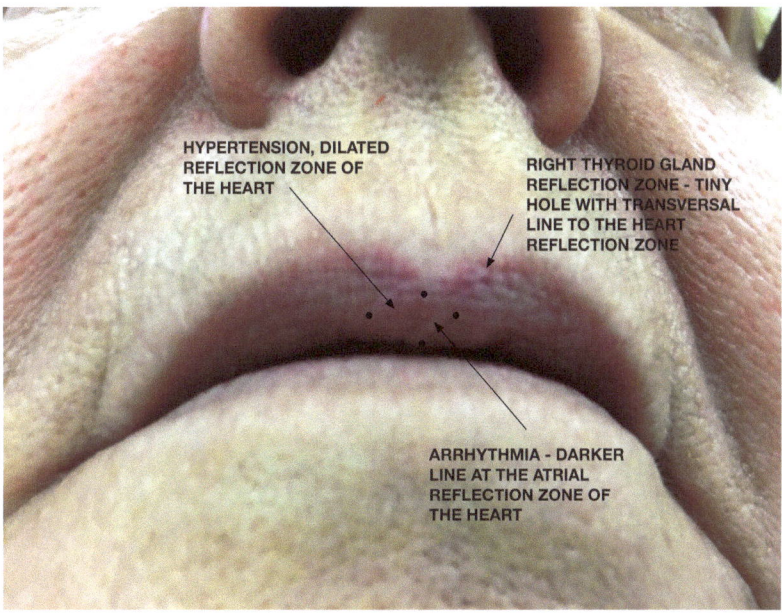

Manifestations of the Diseases on the Lip Organ Zones

Fig. 47 The patient below has been diagnosed with essential hypertension and ventricular arrhythmia. The heart reflection zone is red and dilated (marked by the black points). A red line indicating arrhythmia can be seen on the ventricular reflection zone (arrow).

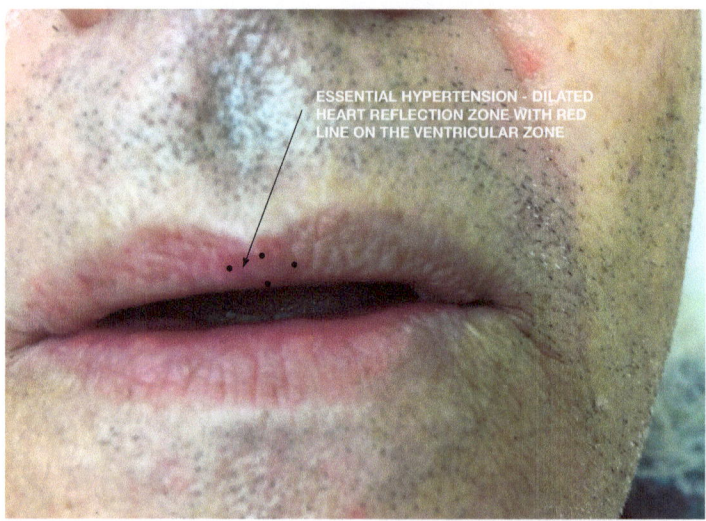

Fig. 48 The photo below is of a patient with renal hypertension, a hypertrophic left ventricle, and kidney pain. The right kidney is more painful than the left kidney. The heart reflection zone is red and swollen (marked by black points). The brown spot reflects the hypertrophic left ventricle (arrow). Within the red kidney reflection zones, the right kidney is more visible than the left kidney, indicative of the level of pain.

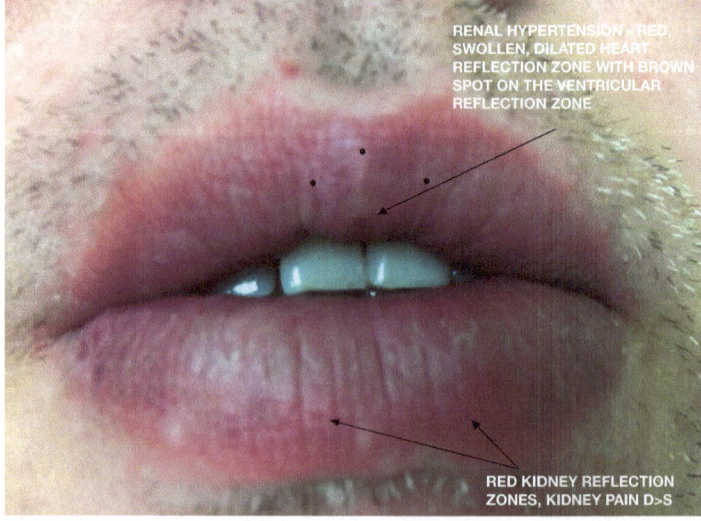

2.2. Hypotension

Patients with hypotension, regardless of the etiology of their disease, have a normal sized or slightly smaller heart reflection zone on the upper lip that is accompanied by a light pink color.

Fig. 49 The patient in the photo below has hypothyroidism and exhibits hypotension, bradicardia, muscular weakness, hair loss, and cold intolerance. The size of the heart reflection zone is little smaller than normal and is of a light pink color (marked by the black points). The patient has long history of hypothyroidism and has used hormonal replacement therapy (Levo Thyroxin), which created atrophy of the thyroid gland represented by replacement of the lip membrane with skin on the thyroid reflection zones.

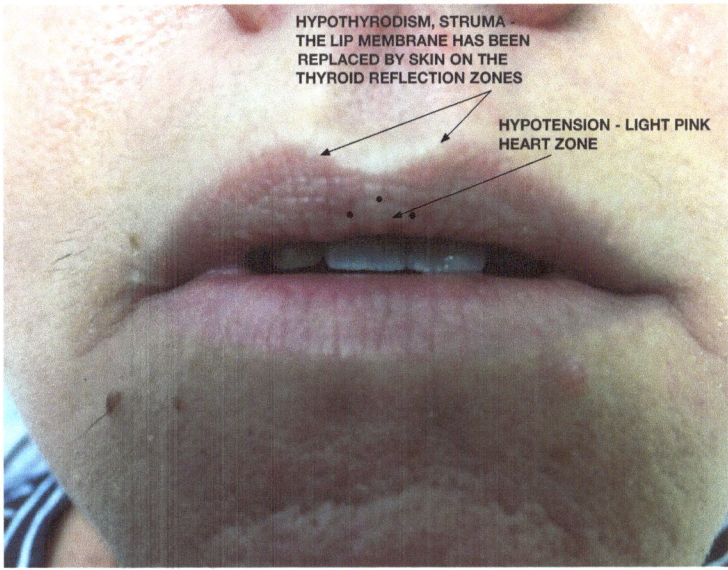

2.3. Arrhythmia

When a patient has supraventricular arrhythmia, the arrhythmia is represented with an angular line on the atrial zone within the heart reflection zone. A line appears on the ventricular reflection zone when a patient has ventricular arrhythmia. In cases where hyperthyroidism is also present, a line forms between the thyroid reflection zone and the heart zone.

Fig. 50 The photo below represents a patient with supraventricular arrhythmia (tachycardia). The heart reflection zone is dilated (marked by the black points). The arrhythmia is indicated by the dark line running through the atrial reflection zone (arrow).

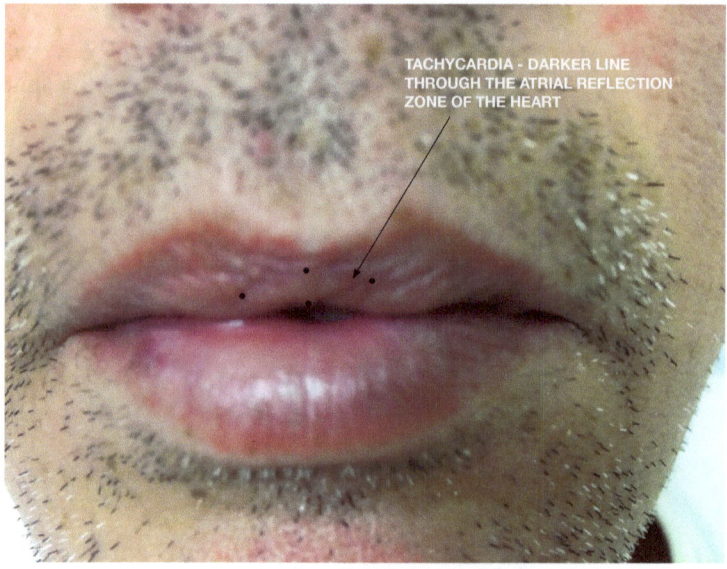

Fig. 51 The patient below has vegetative dystonic syndrome characterized by unstable blood pressure, tachycardia, sweating, anxiety, and insomnia. The heart reflection zone is dilated and swollen (marked by the black points). The arrhythmia can be seen as a line through the atrial reflection zone.

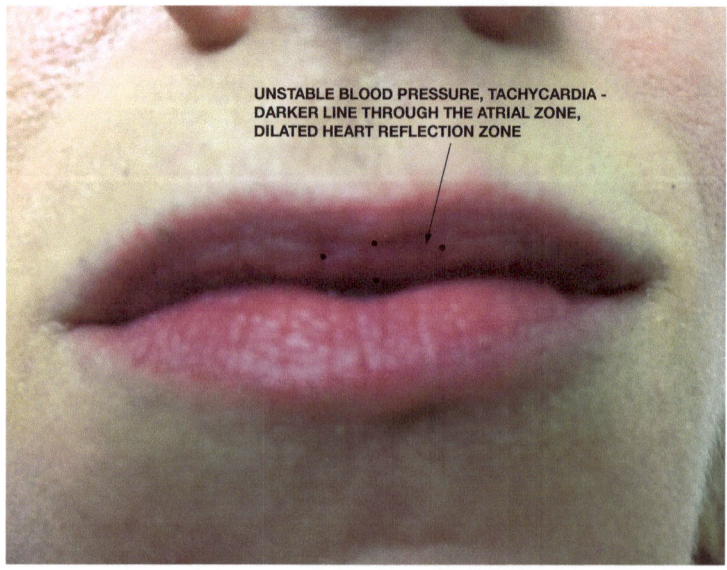

Fig. 52 A photograph of a patient with supraventricular arrhythmia is presented below. A very clear curved line can be seen over the atrial reflection zone. The heart reflection zone is swollen.

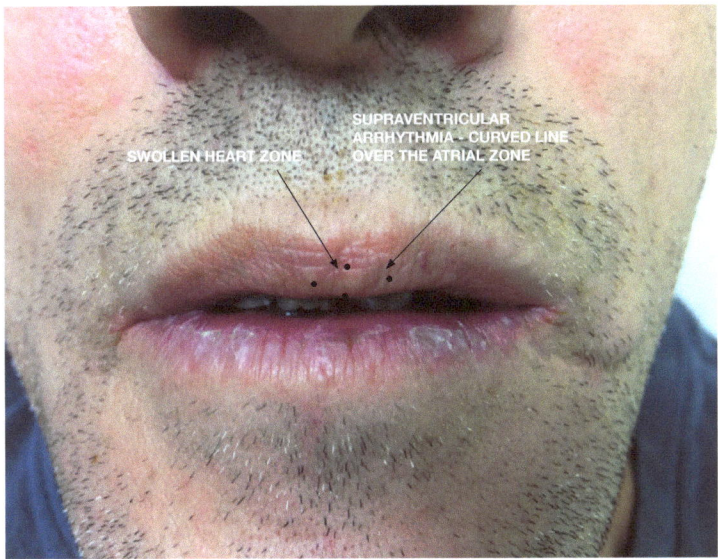

Fig. 53 The photo below is of a patient with supraventricular arrhythmia, which is a consequence of hyperthyroidism. The darker line on the atrial reflection zone connects the atrial zone with the right thyroid reflection zone (shorter arrow). The longer dark line connects the left thyroid reflection zone with the atrial reflection zone (longer arrow). The thyroid reflection zones are slightly reddish.

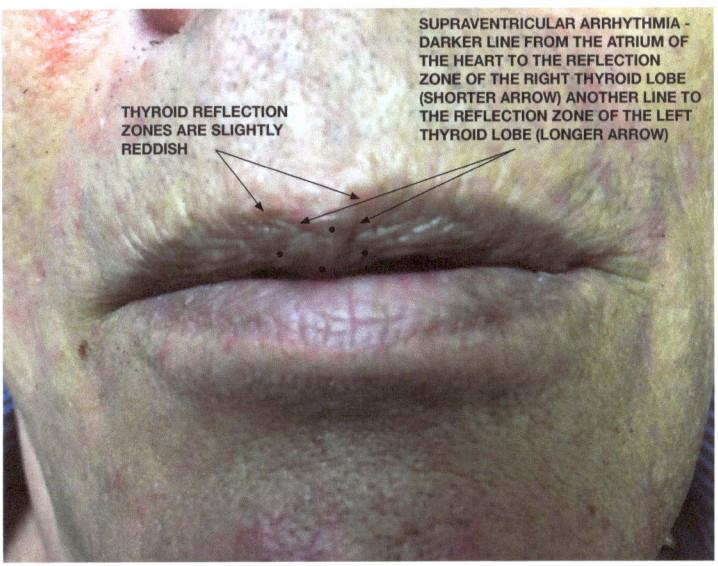

Fig. 54 The patient below has been diagnosed with struma (a swelling of the neck due to an enlarged thyroid gland), hyperthyroidism, supraventricular arrhythmia, and pneumosclerosis. A dark spot and line (marked by the shorter arrow) can be seen on the atrial reflection zone, as can a vertical darker line, which connects the atrial reflection zone with the right thyroid reflection zone (longer arrow).

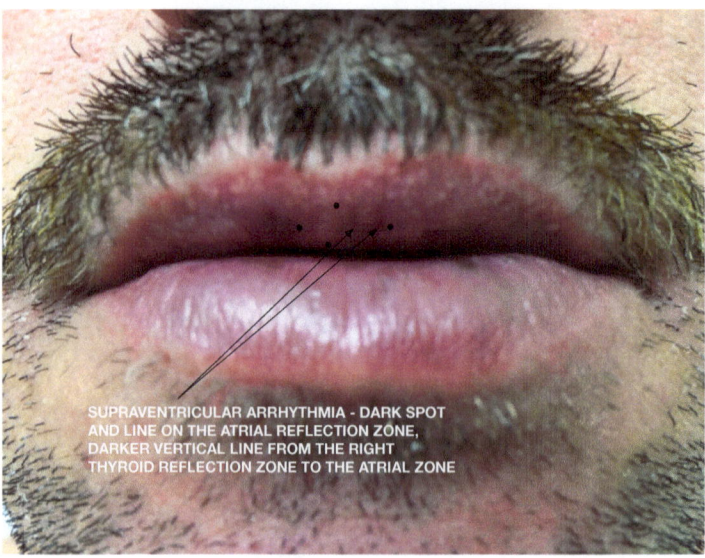

Fig. 55 The photograph below is of a patient with ventricular arrhythmia. The heart reflection zone is slightly dilated and is reddish pink in color (marked by the black points). Arrhythmia is indicated by the dark lines in the ventricular reflection zone, as well as by the small dark spot.

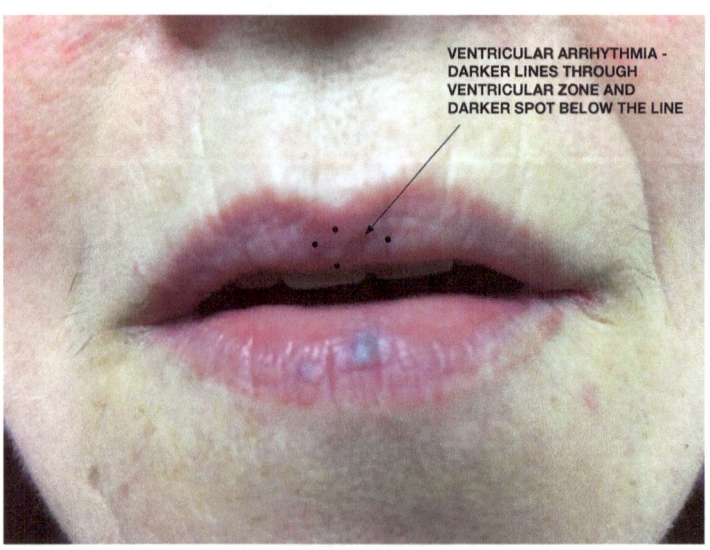

Fig. 56 This patient below has a familial predisposition to heart disease. The patient has been diagnosed with ventricular arrhythmia. The atrial reflection zone contains a dark spot. There is a dark vertical line above the lip. A vertical crack from the ventricular zone has spread to above the lip.

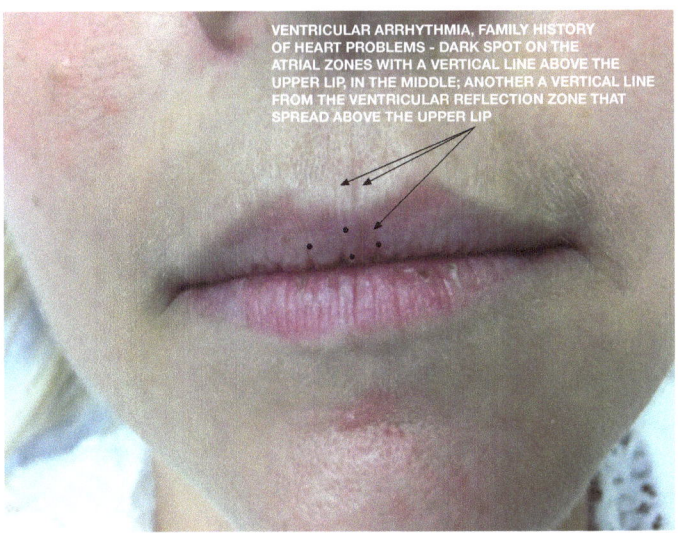

2.4. Heart attack

Fig. 57 The patient below suffered a heart attack three years prior to the date the photograph was taken. The patient has hypertension and dyslipidemia. The heart reflection zone is dilated (marked by the black points). The ventricular reflection zone contains a line and a yellowish bump above the line (arrow).

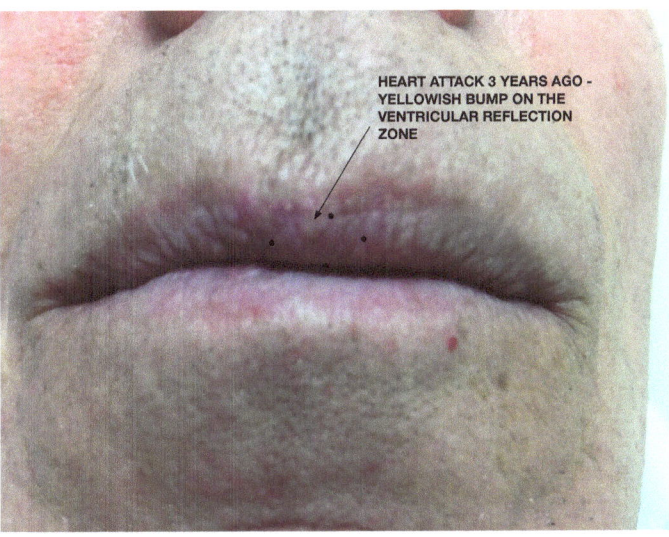

Lip Diagnostics

Fig. 58 The patient in the photograph below had a heart attack three months ago and received two stents to restore the flow of blood to the left descended coronary artery. The heart reflection zone contains a white triangular spot, and the lip projection indicates a heart attack (arrow).

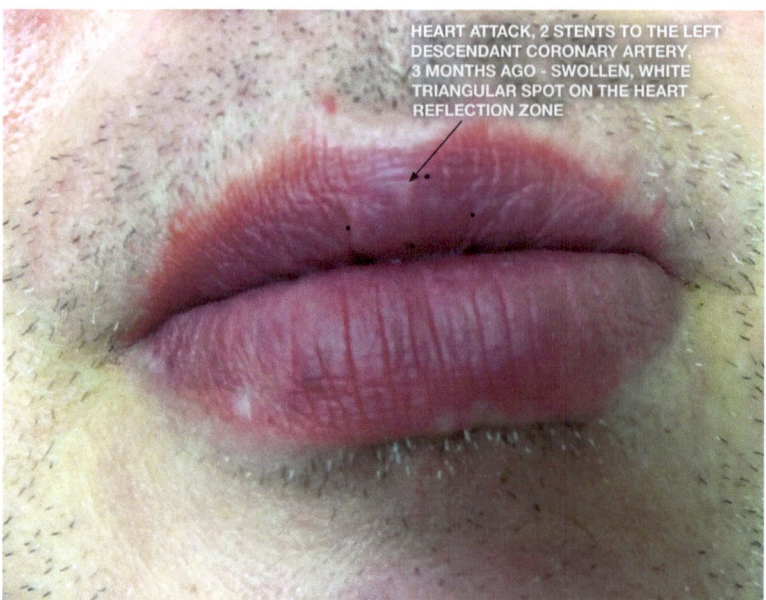

2.5. Heart insufficiency

Patients with heart insufficiency manifest a dilated heart reflection zone, with changes in color. A purplish color indicates blood stasis. Light pink indicates anemia or decreased blood circulation. The color of the heart reflection zone will be the same as the lung reflection zone due to the changed hemodynamic.

Fig. 59 The patient in the photo on next page has mitral and aortic valve prolapse, heart insufficiency, arrhythmia, hypertension, diabetes mellitus, and dyslipidemia. The heart reflection zone is dilated and slightly swollen. An increase in the size of the heart is marked by the black points. The color of the heart, lung, and organ reflection zones on the lower lip is purplish, a manifestation of blood stasis. There is a line on the atrial and ventricular reflection zones that is indicative of arrhythmia (arrows).

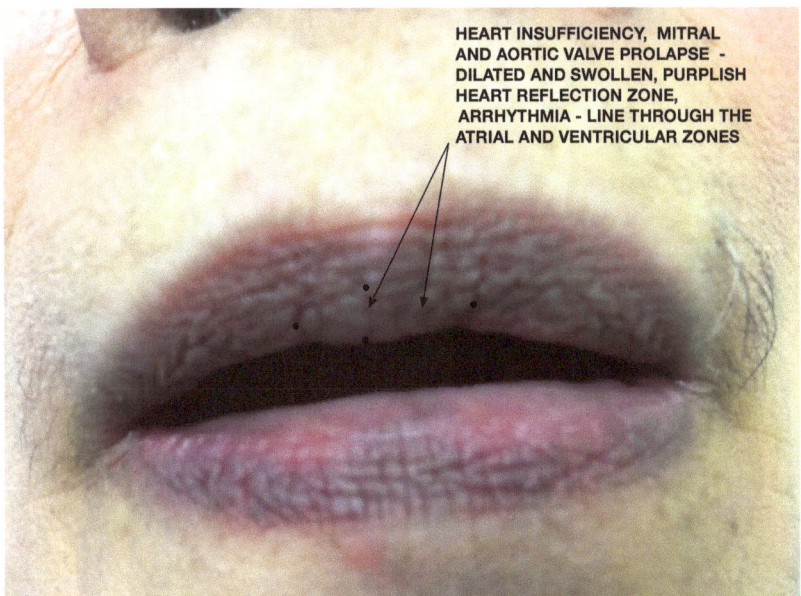

Fig. 60 The patient below has tricuspid, mitral, and aortic valve insufficiency, which lead to cardiomegaly and heart insufficiency. The heart reflection zone is dilated (marked by the black points). The color of the heart reflection zone, and most noticeably of the organ reflection zones on the lower lip, is light pink to white. The atrial, and part of the ventricular, reflection zones are a slightly darker pink because of the changed hemodynamic and regurgitation of the blood through the valves.

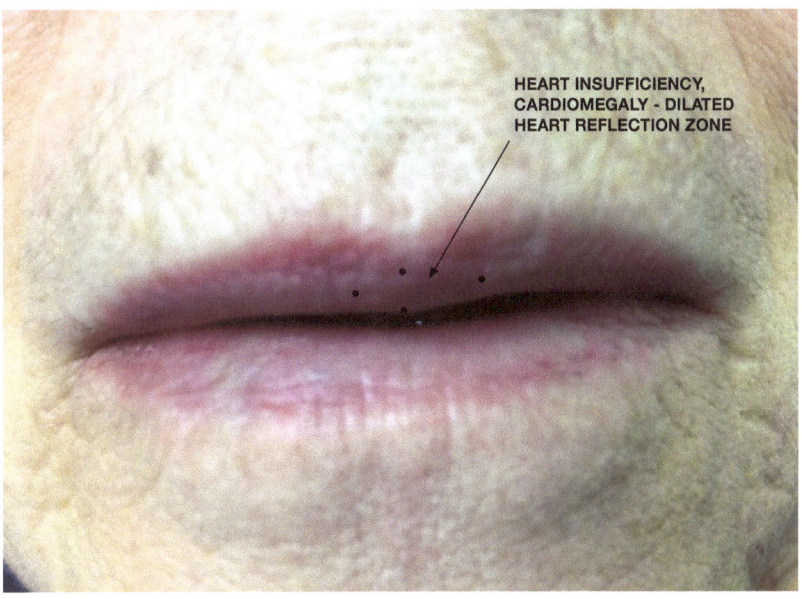

Fig. 61 The photo below is of a patient who has heart insufficiency, arrhythmia, and hypothyroidism. The heart reflection zone is dilated (marked by the black points), and light pink in color. There is a vertical line from the right thyroid reflection zone to the atrial reflection zone due to the influence of the thyroid on the heart rhythm (arrow).

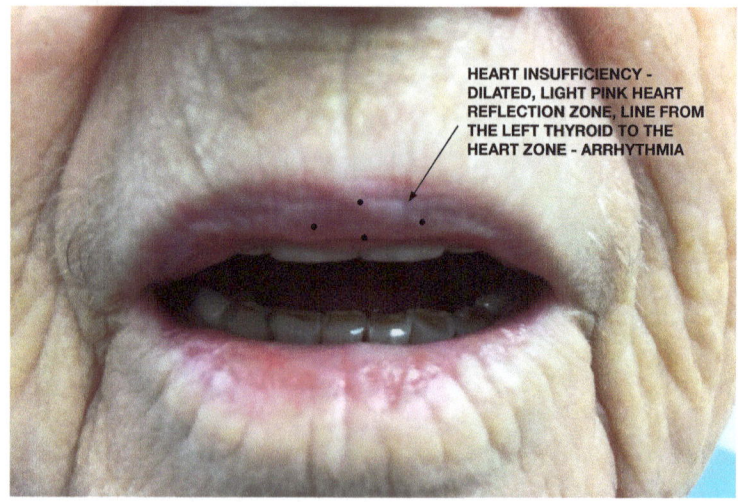

Fig. 62 The patient shown below developed heart insufficiency and arrhythmia after suffering lung cancer and chronic pleurisy. The heart reflection zone is dilated and swollen (marked by the black points). A transversal line that spread to the lung reflection zones can be seen across the heart reflection zone. The atrial reflection zone contains a line that is indicative of arrhythmia (arrow). The color of the heart reflection zone is light pink.

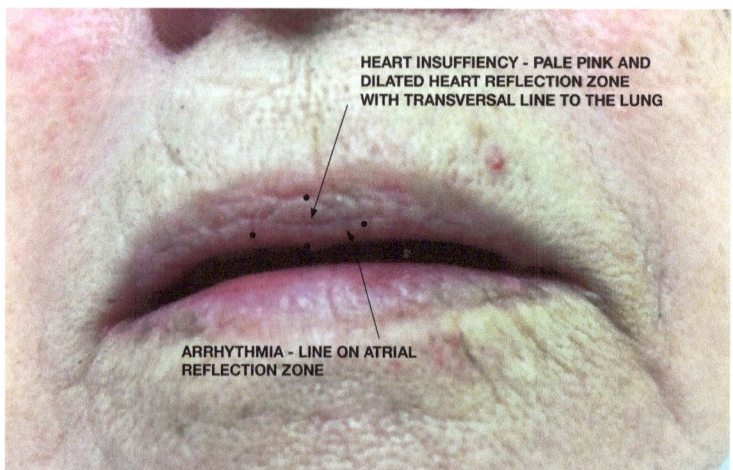

2.6. Valve insufficiency

Fig. 62 The patient below was diagnosed with mitral valve prolapse. She was born with a large cyst on the left lung, which compressed the heart and caused the mitral valve to prolapse. Subsequently, the cyst was surgically removed. A darker spot and a transversal line indicative of the mitral valve prolapse can be seen within the atrial reflection zone (arrow). The left lung reflection zone contains a vertical white line, which ascends to above the upper lip. It developed after the surgical procedure.

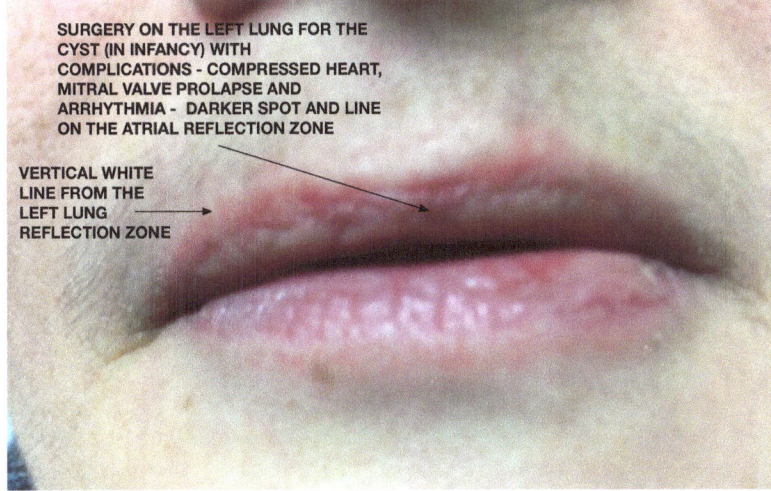

Fig. 63 The patient shown below has an artificial mitral valve. The heart and lung reflection zones are a purplish white color and contain small bumps.

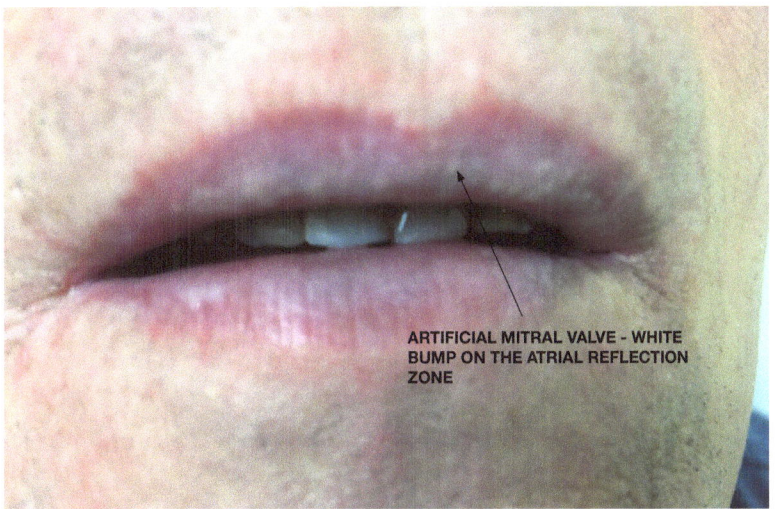

Lip Diagnostics

Fig. 64 The patient shown below has rheumatoid myocarditis, and insufficiency of the tricuspid, mitral, and aortal valves. The heart reflection zone is red, swollen, and dilated (marked by the black points). The atrial and ventricular reflection zones contain lines that developed at an angle (arrows).

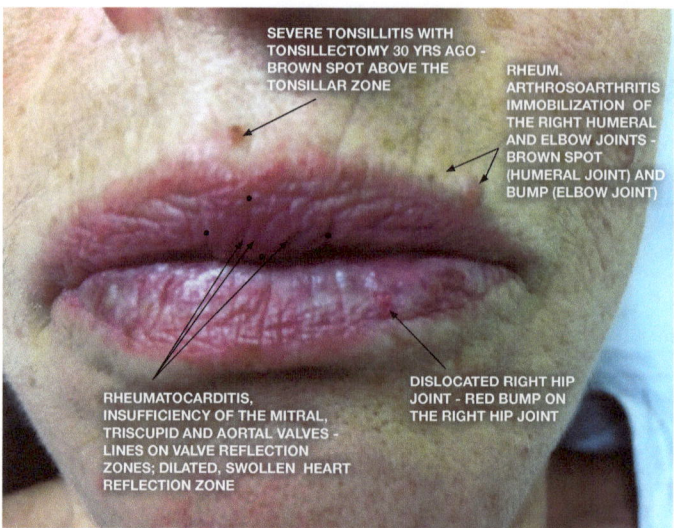

2.7. Varicose veins

Dilated or varicose veins are the result of a weakness in the connective tissue within the walls of a vein, increased blood viscosity, and blood stasis. Varicose veins, depending on the stage of the progression, manifest as purple to brown, slightly swollen spots or lines within the leg reflection zones on the lower lip.

Fig. 65 The photo below is of a patient with varicose veins of the right leg – v. saphenous superficially. There is a purplish line within the right leg reflection zone, just below the right knee (arrow).

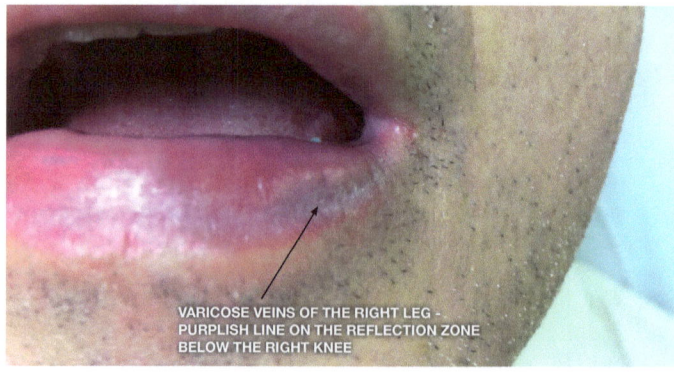

Fig. 66 The patient below has chronic varicose veins of the legs. The reflection zones below the knees contain purplish brown, swollen spots (arrows).

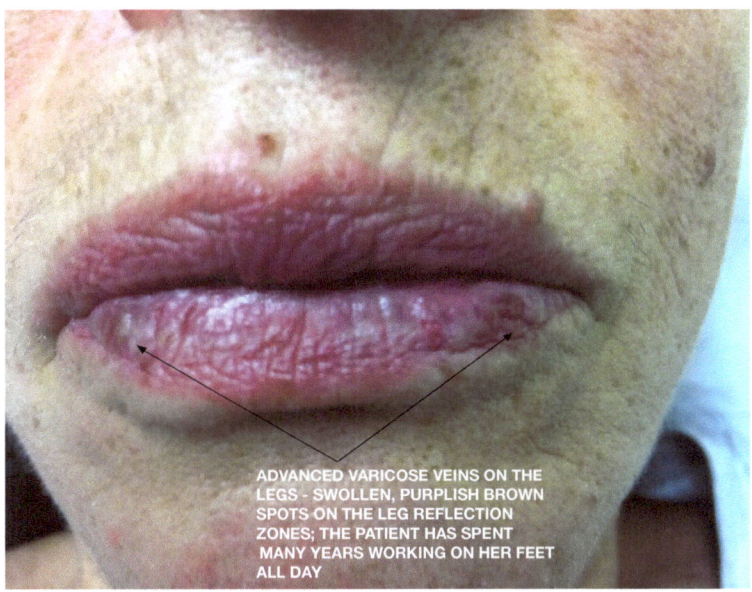

ADVANCED VARICOSE VEINS ON THE LEGS - SWOLLEN, PURPLISH BROWN SPOTS ON THE LEG REFLECTION ZONES; THE PATIENT HAS SPENT MANY YEARS WORKING ON HER FEET ALL DAY

Fig. 67 The patient below has advanced varicose veins and phlebothrombosis of the right leg. The right leg reflection zone contains a light brown line and yellowish spots.

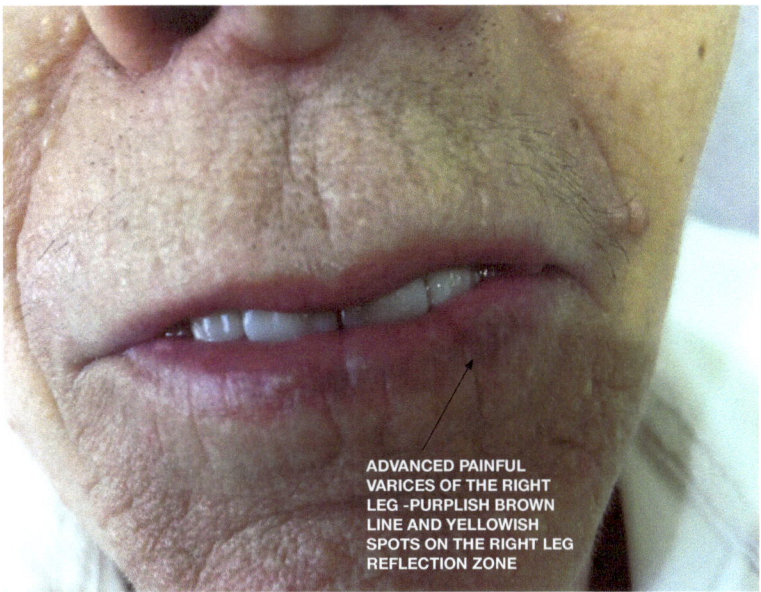

ADVANCED PAINFUL VARICES OF THE RIGHT LEG -PURPLISH BROWN LINE AND YELLOWISH SPOTS ON THE RIGHT LEG REFLECTION ZONE

Lip Diagnostics

2.7. Lymphadenitis

Fig. 68 The patient below has a skin infection of the right axillary region, which caused an infection of the lymph nodes and vasculature of the elbow. The reflection zone of the right arm, from the axillary to the elbow regions, is swollen and light pinkish in color (arrows). The swollen right arm can be seen reflected in the drooping lower rim of the upper lip.

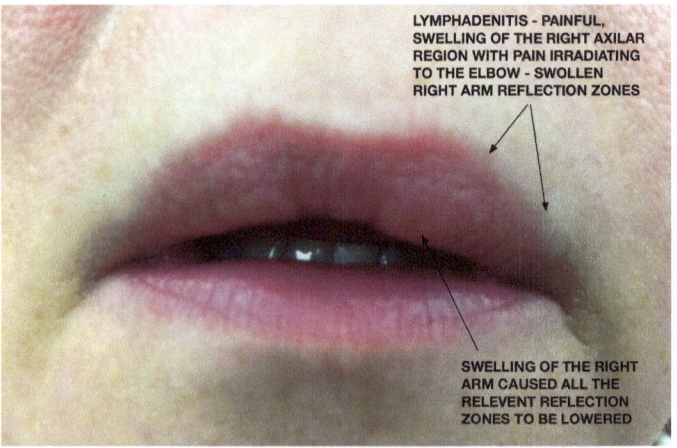

3. Pathologic processes at the gastrointestinal system

3.1. Gastritis. Stomach Ulcer

Fig. 68 The patient below is experiencing nausea, vomiting, heartburn, pain in the stomach region, as well as diarrhea. The patient has been working with toxins for fourteen years. The stomach reflection zone is red in color (marked by the black points). A red spot appears on the liver reflection zone. The white bumps are shown on the descending colon and the rectal reflection zones (arrows at the left side).

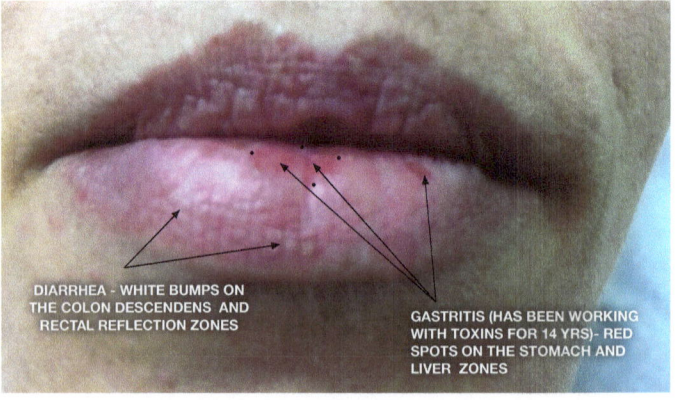

Fig. 68 The patient below has chronic gastritis and enterocolitis, gluten intolerance, and hepatitis type B. The stomach and small intestine reflection zones (marked by the black points) are reddish. The large intestine and liver reflection zones are light pink to white in color (arrows). The stomach and descending colon reflection zones have a slightly decreased turgor. There is a vertical crack through the stomach reflection zone.

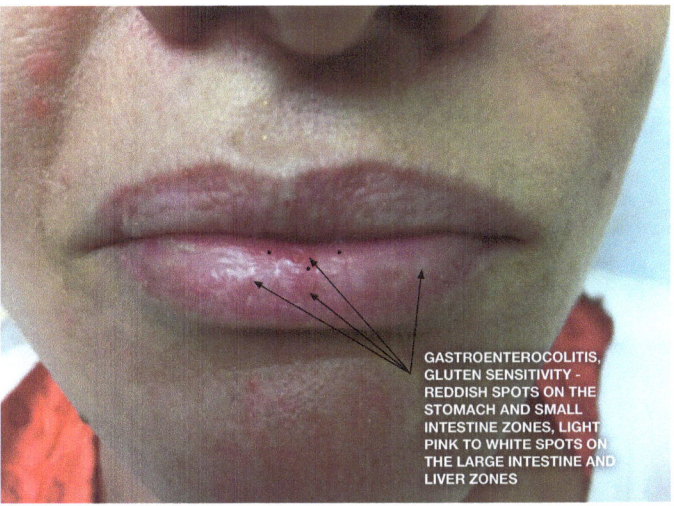

GASTROENTEROCOLITIS, GLUTEN SENSITIVITY - REDDISH SPOTS ON THE STOMACH AND SMALL INTESTINE ZONES, LIGHT PINK TO WHITE SPOTS ON THE LARGE INTESTINE AND LIVER ZONES

Fig. 69 The patient below has been diagnosed with acute gastroenterocolitis, with upper and lower dyspeptic syndrome. She is experiencing severe pain in various parts of the abdomen, along with nausea, vomiting, increased peristalsis, and diarrhea. The reflection zones of the stomach, intestines, pancreas, and liver are swollen and red.

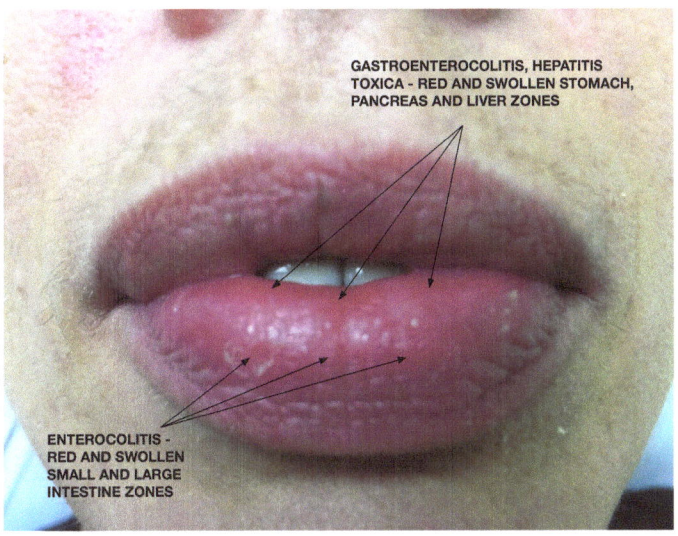

GASTROENTEROCOLITIS, HEPATITIS TOXICA - RED AND SWOLLEN STOMACH, PANCREAS AND LIVER ZONES

ENTEROCOLITIS - RED AND SWOLLEN SMALL AND LARGE INTESTINE ZONES

Lip Diagnostics

Fig. 70 The patient below has been diagnosed with obsessive-compulsive disorder. He is experiencing panic attacks, anxiety, and psychosomatic gastritis characterized by stomachache, nausea, vomiting, and heartburn. The reflection zones on the lower lip are swollen and red. The stomach reflection zone contains a dark reddish spot. The reflection zones of the brain (shorter arrow), thyroid, and lungs are light pink to white. The heart reflection zone contains a darker pink spot (longer arrow).

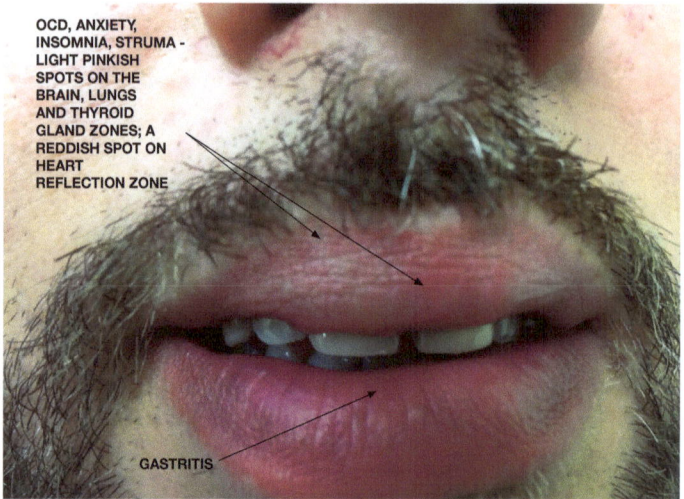

Fig. 71 The patient below has chronic gastritis, cholecystitis, a gall bladder polyp, and a stomach ulcer. She is experiencing pain in the stomach region on an empty stomach, painful right hypochondria, heartburn, nausea, and vomiting. The stomach and gall bladder reflection zones contain red spots. The stomach reflection zone contains a vertical red crack that indicates the ulcer (arrow).

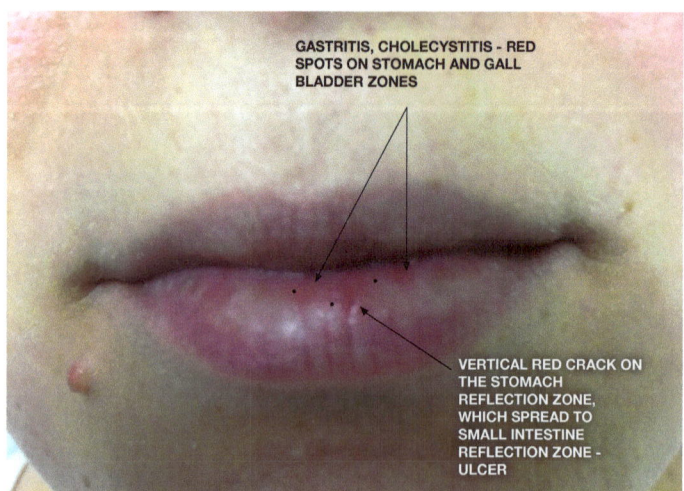

Fig. 72 The patient below has a stomach ulcer and chronic, erosive gastritis accompanied by stomachache, acid regurgitation, and nausea. The stomach reflection zone is red in color and contains a vertical crack (arrow).

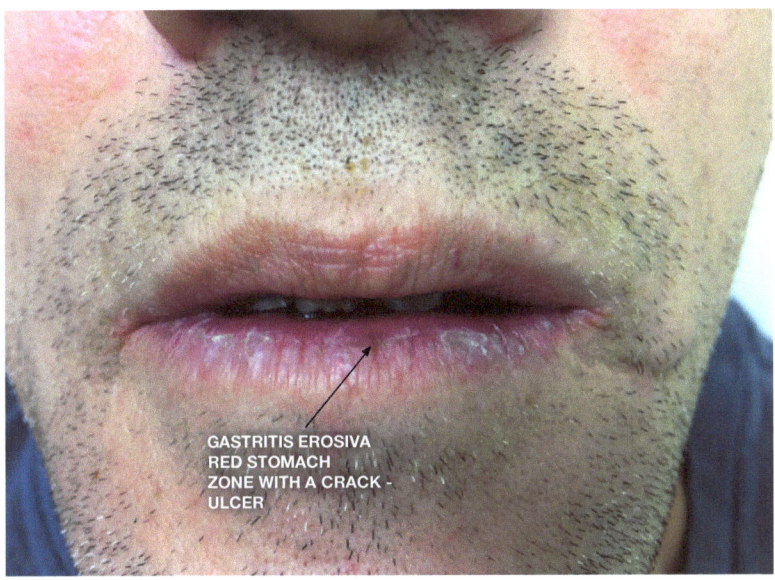

Fig. 73 The photo below is of a patient after surgery for a stab wound in the region of the stomach, duodenum, and pancreas. The patient has chronic pain in the epigastric region. The stomach and duodenum reflection zones contain red spots that are connected with a red line. The pancreatic reflection zone contains a white line.

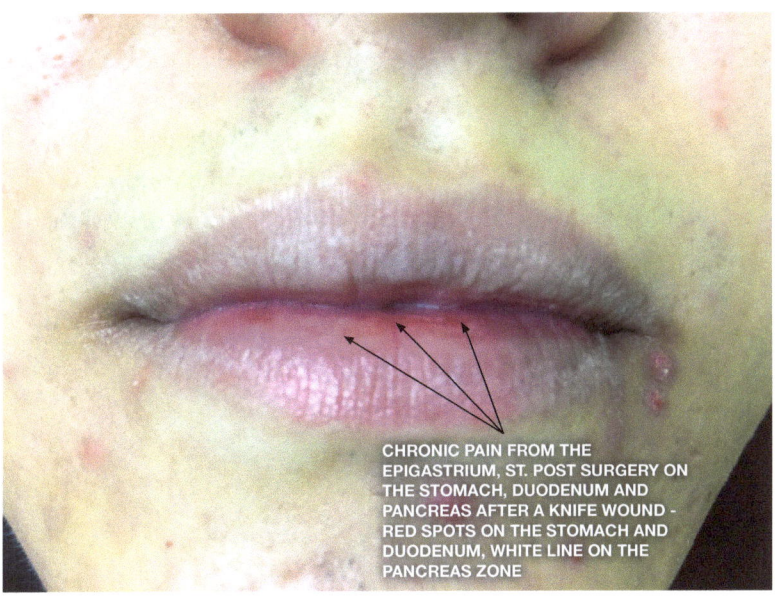

Lip Diagnostics

Fig. 74 The photograph below is of a patient after surgery for a tumor on the left side of the tongue. The tongue reflection zone has a white spot, which signals the location of the tumor (arrow).

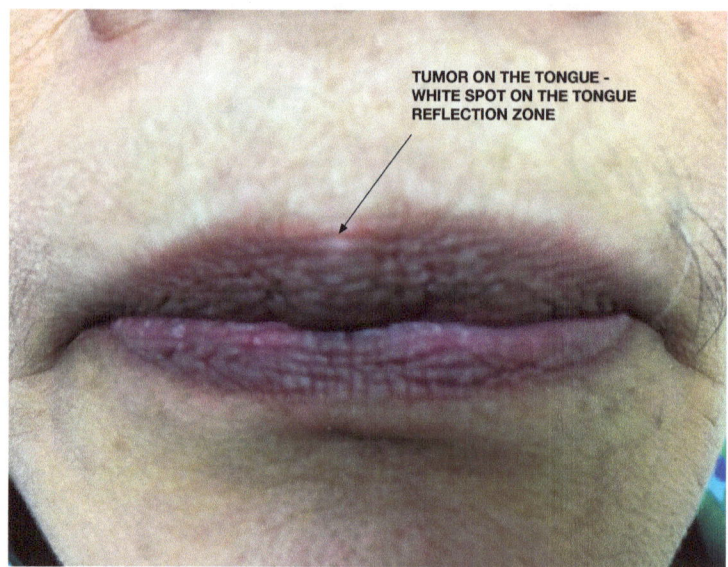

3.2. Enteritis

Fig. 75 The patient in the photograph below has autoimmune enteritis due to gluten intolerance, in addition to anemia. The reflection zones of the intestines contain red and white spots (arrows). At the age of twelve, the patient had heavy eczema. As a side effect of the therapy, the patient developed Stevens-Johnson syndrome. A yellowish bump has formed on the right lumbosacral skin reflection zone (arrow) after the therapy. Stevens-Johnson syndrome is a rare, serious skin disorder most frequently caused by drug sensitivity reaction or an infection, according to Mayo Clinic. In Stevens-Johnson syndrome, the top layer of the skin blisters, peels, and sheds over large areas of the body, potentially even on the inside of the mouth and eyes. Stevens-Johnson syndrome is considered a medical emergency that requires immediate treatment.

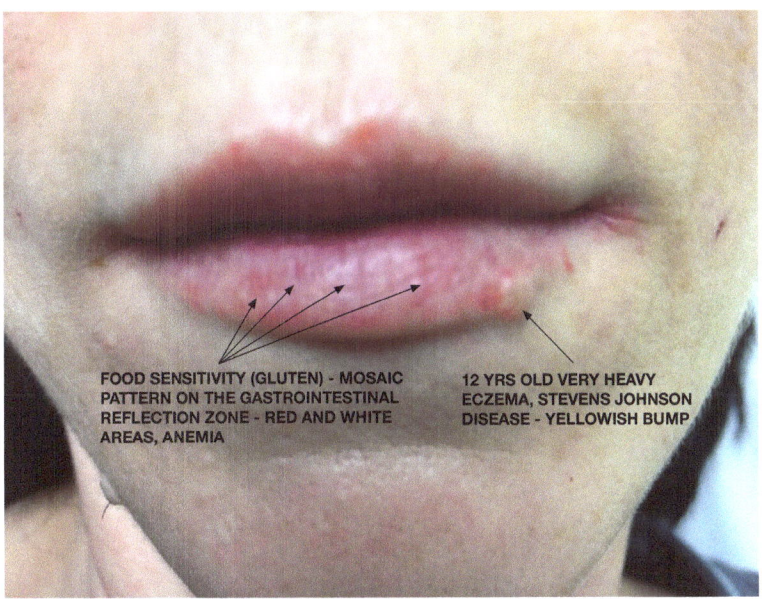

Fig. 76 The patient below has infectious gastroenterocolitis characterized by nausea, vomiting, diarrhea, cramps, and pain in the gastrointestinal tract. A mosaic pattern comprised of white and red dots developed on the swollen reflection zones of the stomach and intestines (arrows). There are very small white bumps on the intestinal zones.

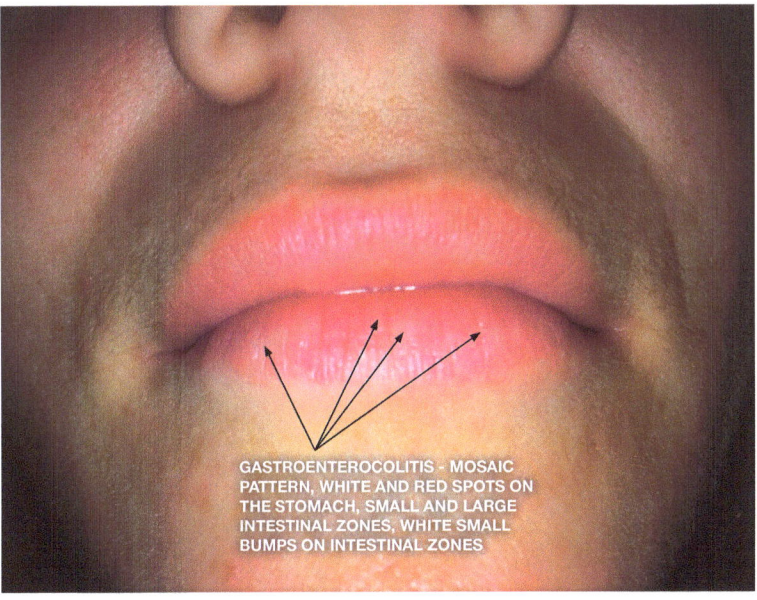

Lip Diagnostics

Fig. 77 The photo below is of a patient with a food allergy, which has manifested as gastroenterocolitis and an allergic skin reaction. The stomach reflection zone contains a vertical central crack and the intestinal reflection zones contain a mosaic pattern characterized by multiple yellowish to white and pink to red spots in an irregular arrangement. A similar mosaic pattern of yellowish and pinkish spots can be seen on the skin reflection zones. The intestinal reflection zones are slightly swollen.

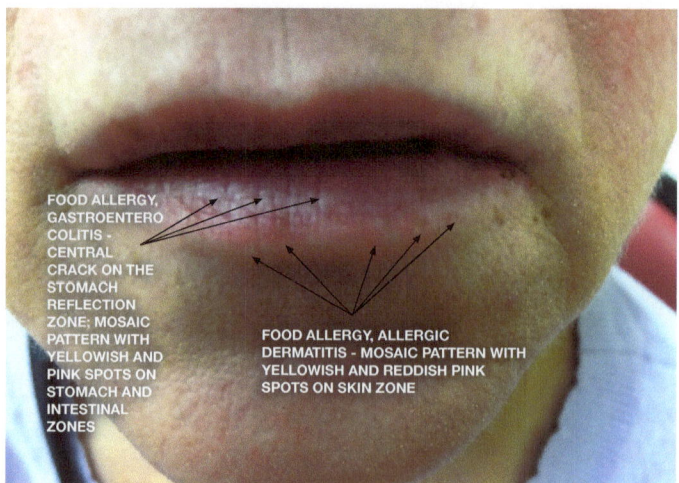

Fig. 78 The photo below is of a patient with a food allergy and chronic gastroenterocolitis. The stomach reflection zone is reddish in color. The intestinal reflection zones are swollen and contain mosaic patterns with yellowish and pinkish spots. The patient has gall bladder stones (cholelithyasis). There is a reddish line through the gall bladder reflection zone on the lower lip.

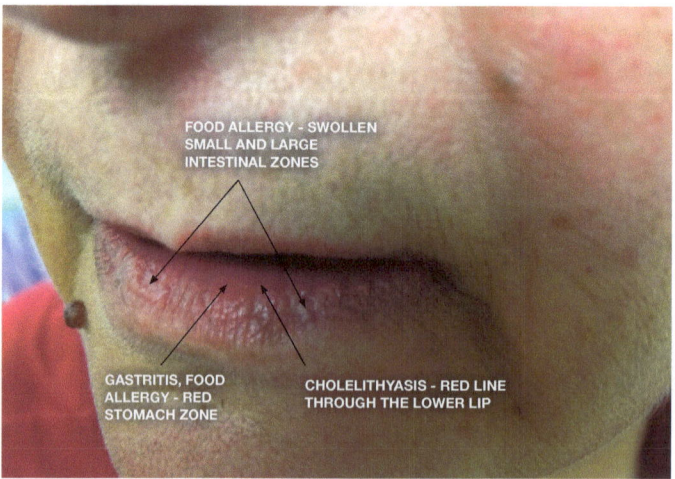

Manifestations of the Diseases on the Lip Organ Zones

3.3. Colitis

Irritation to the colon membrane can come from pathologic microorganisms e.g. bacteria, virus, fungus; autoimmune processes, such as Crohn's disease; infectious colitis; or various kinds of toxins (professional and domestic, pesticides in food, medications, or metabolic toxins).

A. Colitis from a bacterial infection

Fig. 79 The patient below has acute colitis characterized by diarrhea, pain, and cramps in the abdominal region, in addition to blood and mucus in the stool. The colon reflection zones are swollen and red in color.

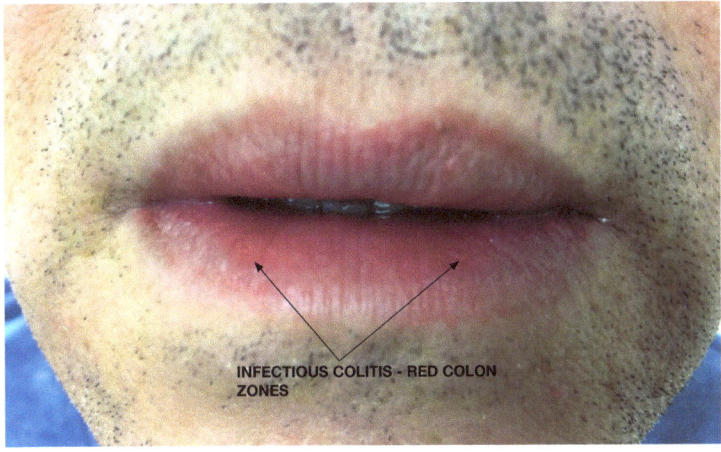

Fig. 80 The patient shown below has an acute infection of the rectum (proctitis). The rectal reflection zone contains a red spot with a peeling membrane.

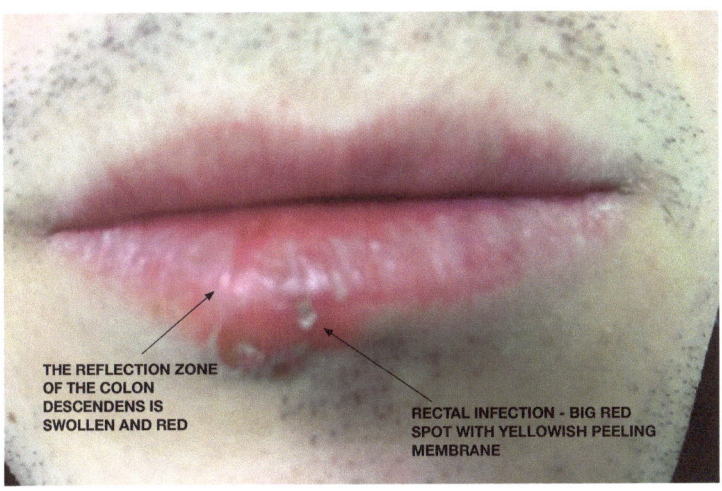

Fig. 81 The patient below has chronic colitis. The reflection zones of the small and large intestines are dry, and swollen. The peeling membranes are light pink in color. Many vertical cracks can be seen in the small and large intestinal reflection zones.

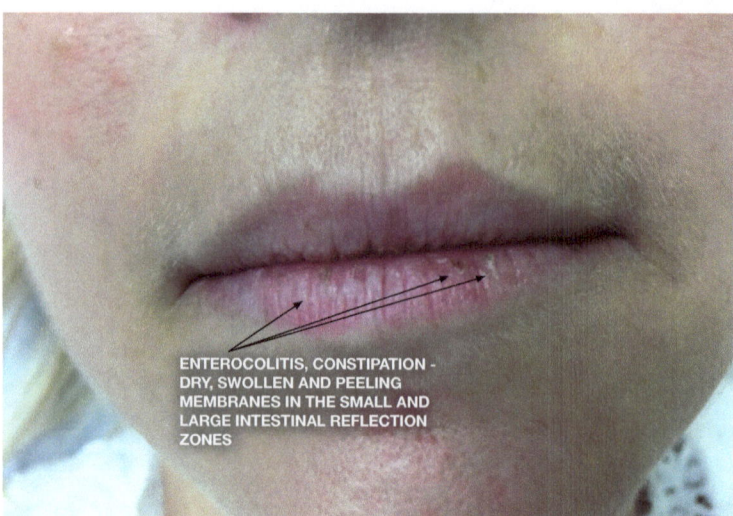

ENTEROCOLITIS, CONSTIPATION - DRY, SWOLLEN AND PEELING MEMBRANES IN THE SMALL AND LARGE INTESTINAL REFLECTION ZONES

B. Autoimmune colitis

Fig. 82 The patient below has had ulcerative colitis since the age of ten. The patient periodically experiences episodes of pain, cramps, and diarrhea with blood and mucus. The colon reflection zone is swollen and reddish pink. The reflection zones of the spleen, pancreas, and liver are swollen as well.

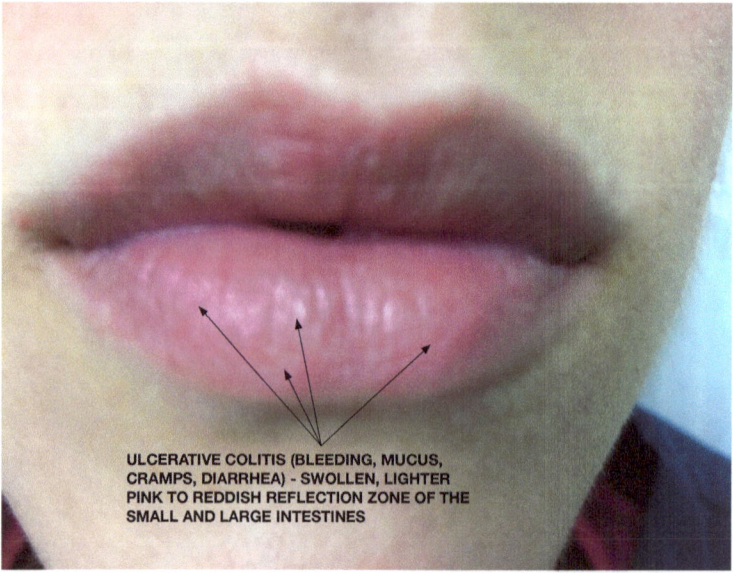

ULCERATIVE COLITIS (BLEEDING, MUCUS, CRAMPS, DIARRHEA) - SWOLLEN, LIGHTER PINK TO REDDISH REFLECTION ZONE OF THE SMALL AND LARGE INTESTINES

Fig. 83 The patient below has an autoimmune process in the ascendant part of the colon (Crohn`s disease). The ascendant and ileocecal region of the colon are swollen and red in color.

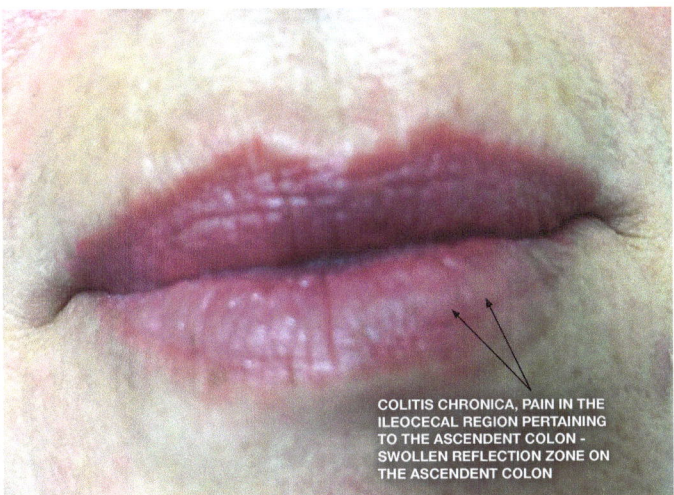

COLITIS CHRONICA, PAIN IN THE ILEOCECAL REGION PERTAINING TO THE ASCENDENT COLON - SWOLLEN REFLECTION ZONE ON THE ASCENDENT COLON

C. Toxic colitis

Fig. 84 The patient in the photograph below works with professional toxins (paints). He has developed toxic gastroenterocolitis, toxic hepatitis, dyslipidemia, and hemorrhoids. The reflection zones of the stomach, liver, small and large intestines are swollen. The stomach and liver reflection zones are light pink in color. The small and large intestine reflection zones are light yellowish to white. The borders of the intestinal reflection zones are marked with brown lines.

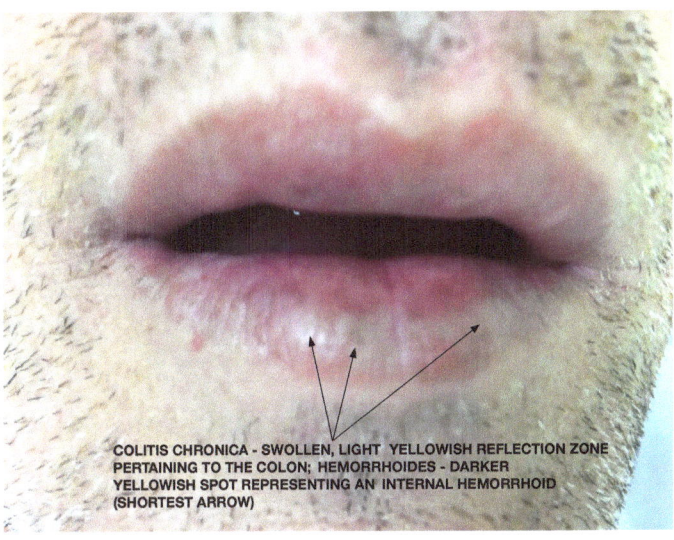

COLITIS CHRONICA - SWOLLEN, LIGHT YELLOWISH REFLECTION ZONE PERTAINING TO THE COLON; HEMORRHOIDES - DARKER YELLOWISH SPOT REPRESENTING AN INTERNAL HEMORRHOID (SHORTEST ARROW)

Lip Diagnostics

Fig. 85 The patient below developed toxic hemorrhagic colitis after therapy with clyndamycin. The large intestine reflection zone is purplish red in color. The reflection zone of the descending colon is swollen.

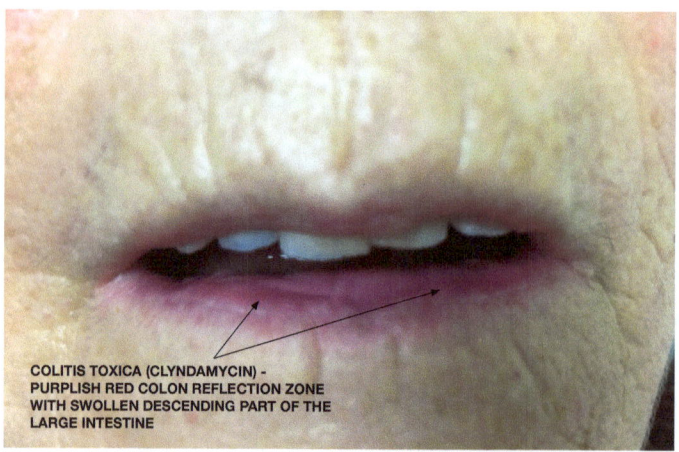

D. Polyps and Diverticulosis of the Colon

Fig. 86 The patient below was diagnosed with cancer of the appendix, lymphadenitis in the right inguinal region, polyps in the ascendant colon (ectomated), diverticulosis in the sigmoid section of the colon, hemorrhoids, and hypothyroidism. The stomach, small, and large intestine reflection zones are light pink in color and are slightly swollen. The illeocecal reflection zone is dilated and is even more swollen than other parts of the gastrointestinal refection zone. A brown spot has formed in the zone of the ectomated polyp on the ascendant colon (arrow). Two brown points, signifying polyps, have formed within the sigmoid reflection zone. The three white bumps indicate diverticulosis (arrows).

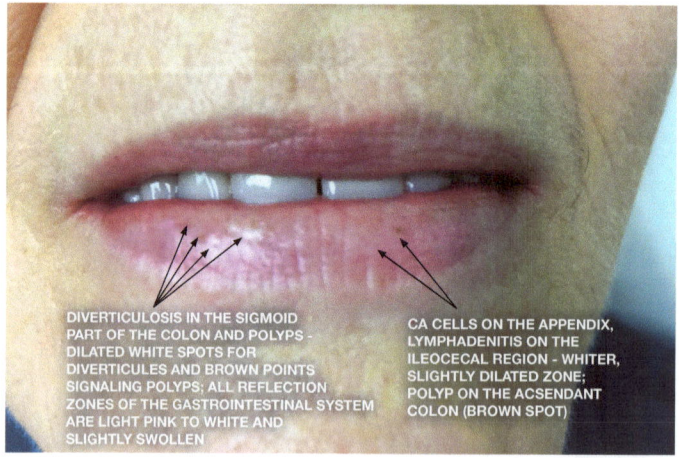

Manifestations of the Diseases on the Lip Organ Zones

Fig. 87 The photo of the patient below was taken immediately after a polypectomy of the colon descendens colon. Three bumps have formed in the reflection zone of the colon descendens (arrows). Later the bumps will be replaced with brown spots.

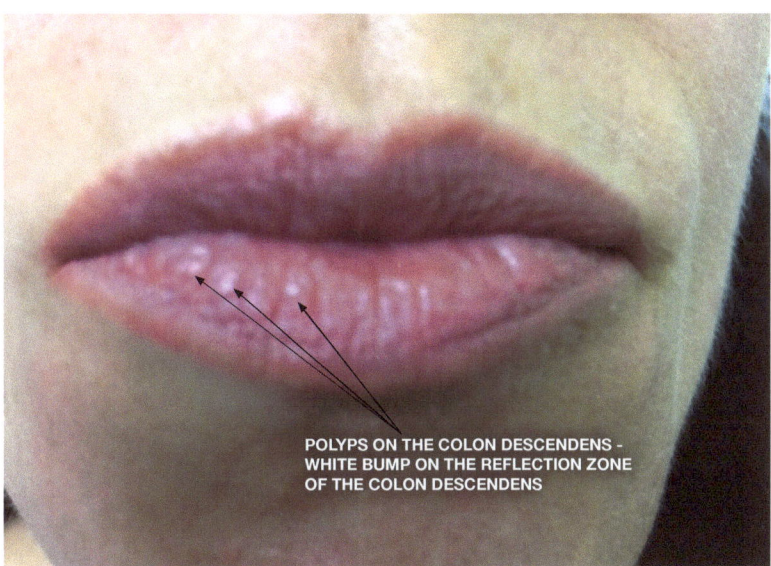

Fig. 88 The patient below had surgery for hemorrhoids. The reflection zone of the anus and lower part of the rectum, located a little to the left of the middle line on the lower lip, contains two white spots (arrows).

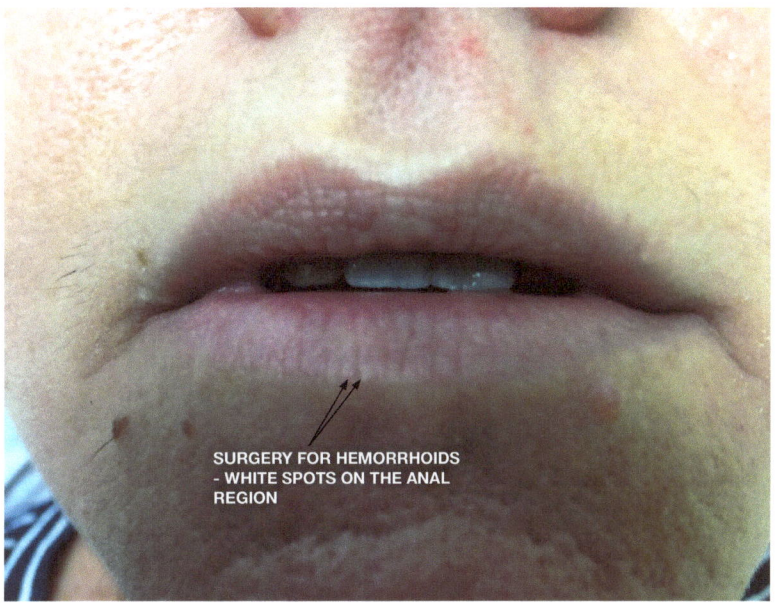

3.4. Hepatitis. Cirrhosis

A. Infectious Hepatitis

Fig. 89 The patient pictured below contracted hepatitis type A during childhood. The liver reflection zone is purplish black in color.

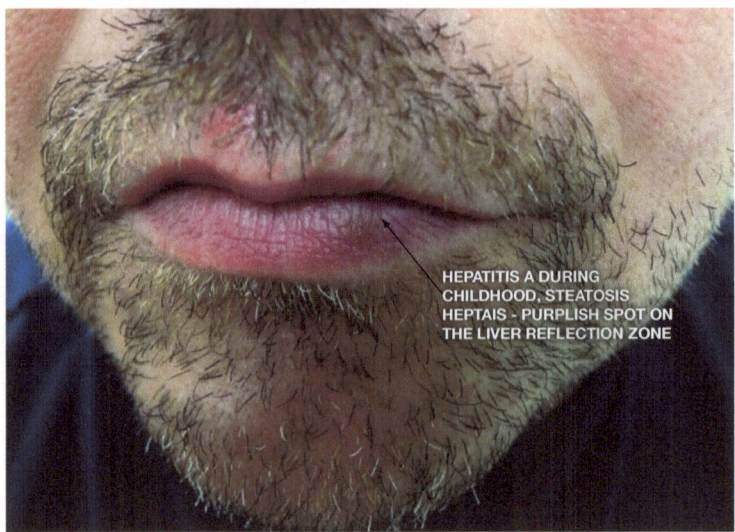

Fig. 90 The patient below has chronic hepatitis type B with increased transaminases. The liver reflection zone contains a mosaic pattern comprised of red, white, and pink spots.

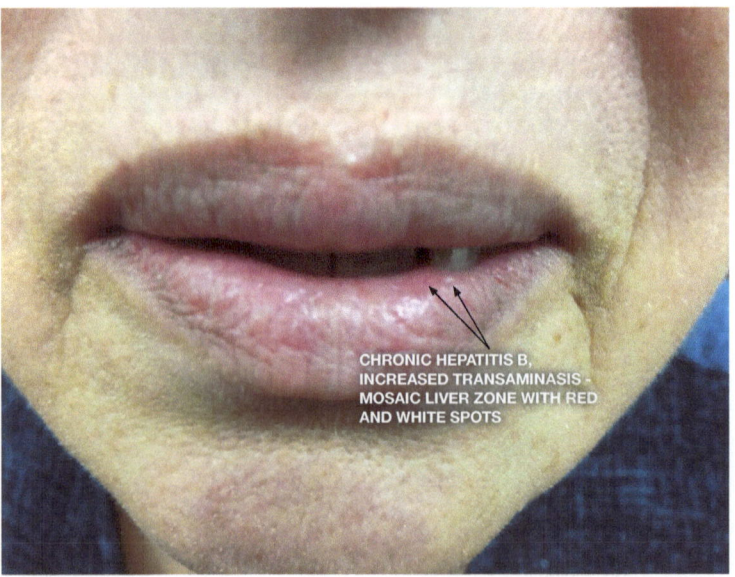

Fig. 91 The patient below has been diagnosed with chronic hepatitis type B, leukocytosis, and psoriasis. The liver reflection zone contains a mosaic pattern comprised of purplish and yellowish spots. The lower lip is flat and smooth.

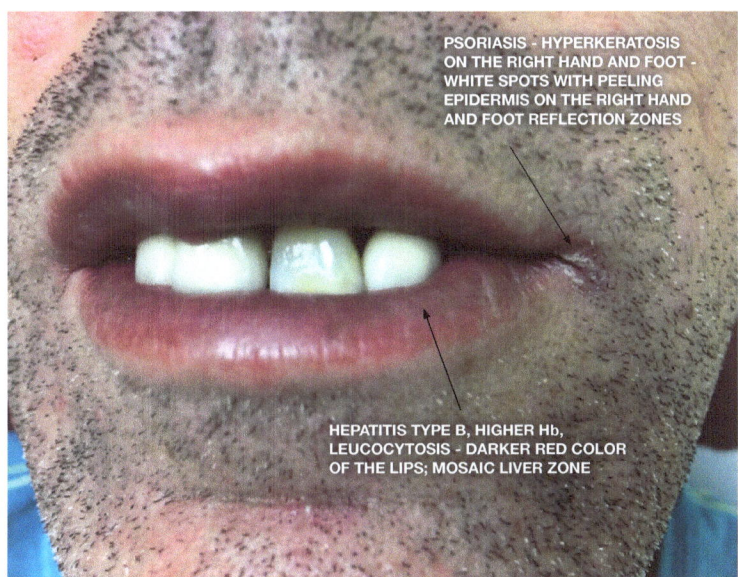

Fig. 92 The patient below has hepatitis type C, increased transaminases, and gastritis. The liver and spleen reflection zones are swollen. The liver reflection zone contains a mosaic pattern comprised of white, red, and pink spots. The stomach reflection zone is light pinkish in color and contains a red spot.

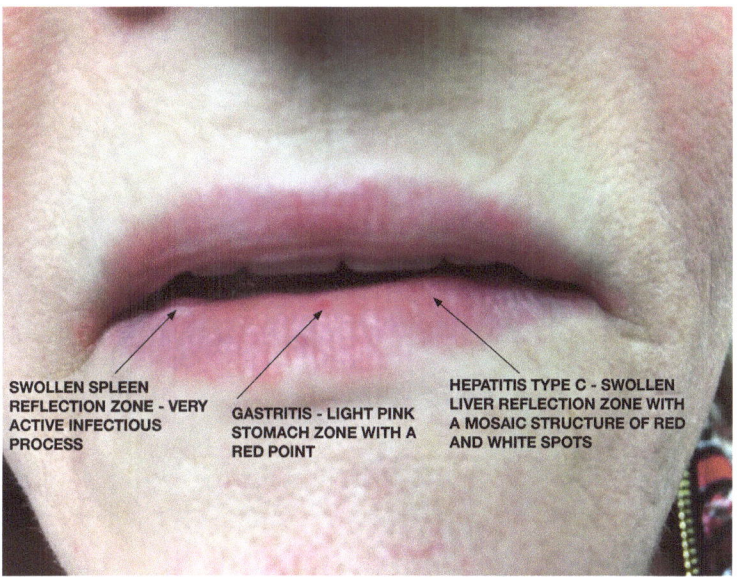

B. Cirrhosis

Fig. 93 The patient below has been diagnosed with primary biliary cirrhosis. The spleen and liver reflection zones are swollen. The liver reflection zone is light pink in color and contains a central red spot.

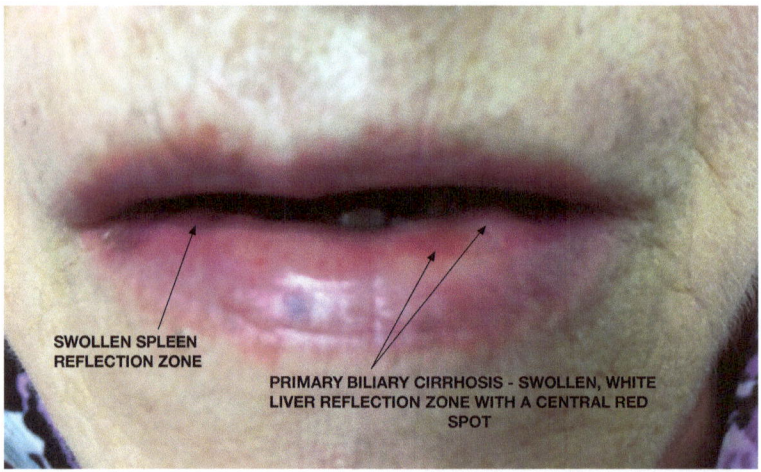

Fig. 94.1-2 The patient pictured below has chronic hepatitis type C, cirrhosis, and diabetes mellitus. The liver reflection zone is swollen and reduced in size. It is light pink in color and the white and red spots on it form a mosaic pattern. The pancreatic reflection zone contains a white vertical line through the lower lip indicating diabetes mellitus.

Fig. 94.1

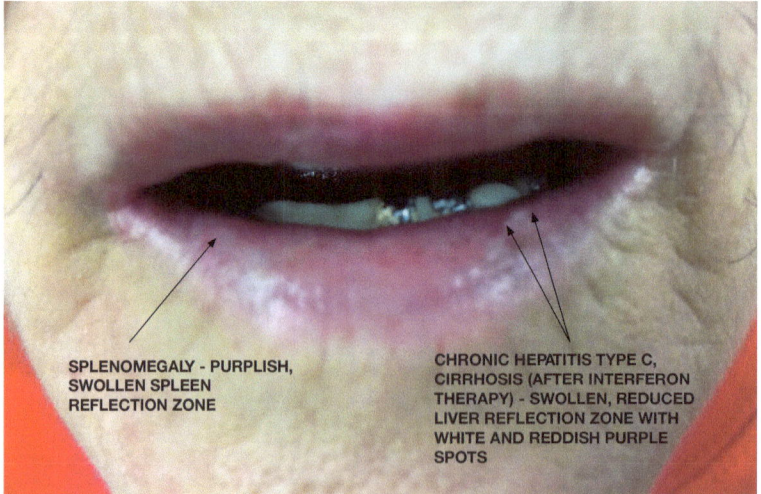

Fig. 94.2

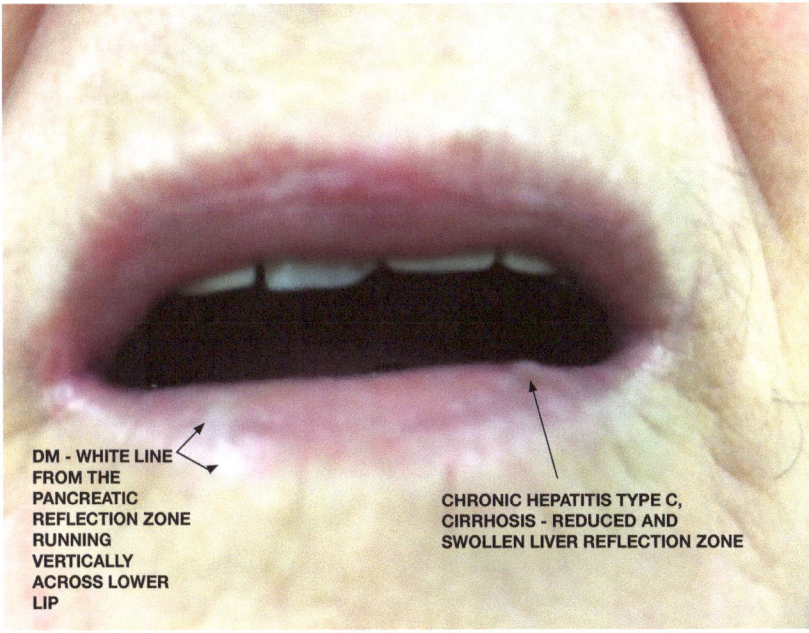

Fig. 95 The patient below has cirrhosis, a decreased number of erythrocytes, a low white blood count, decreased platelets, and increased bilirubin. The liver reflection zone is flat, shiny, a bit depressed, and light pink to reddish in color.

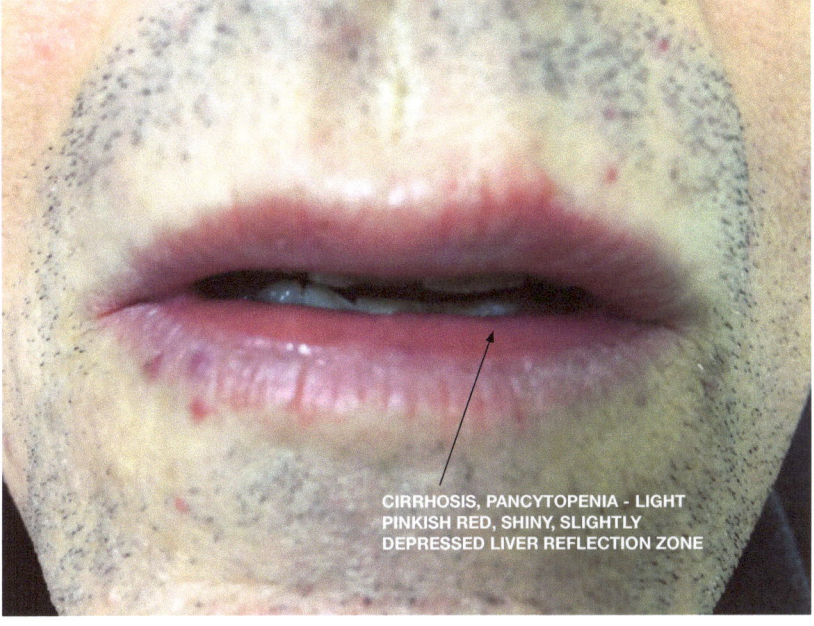

C. Toxic hepatitis

Fig. 96 The patient in the photograph below developed toxic hepatitis after imbibing stimulating beverages. The lip membrane is smooth and tight with red vertical cracks on the liver, gall bladder, stomach, and pancreatic reflection zones (arrows). There is a vertical fold from the liver zone through the lower lip. Another transversal fold has formed from the descending part of the colon and through the small intestine zone to the liver reflection zone. The reflection zones of the liver, stomach, and pancreas contain light pink and red spots.

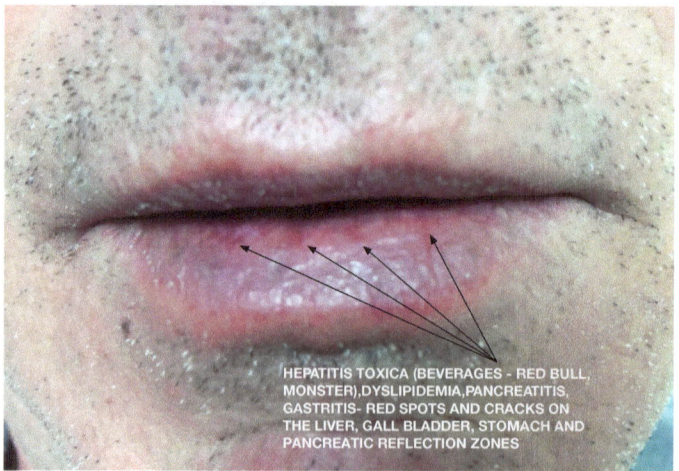

Fig. 97 The patient below, who has been diagnosed with toxic hepatitis, was exposed to construction materials such as paints, varnishes, dust, and alcohol for many years. Two vertical black lines can be seen in the liver reflection zone (arrows).

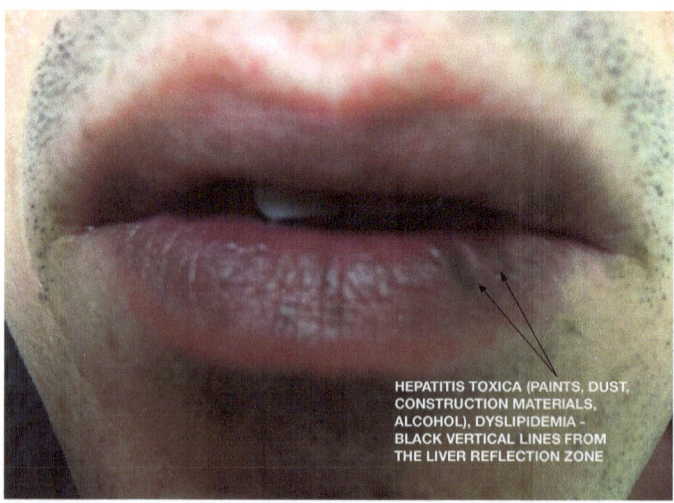

Fig. 98 The patient below contracted toxic hepatitis from drinking alcohol. The liver reflection zone shows decreased turgor; a white, peeling membrane; and purple, yellowish, and pink spots.

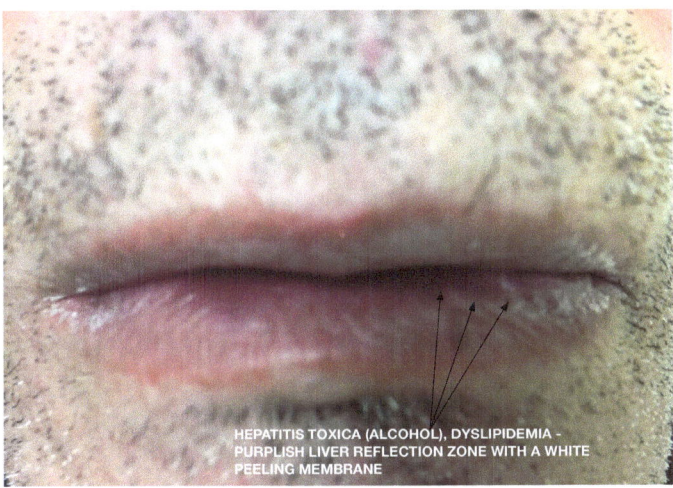

HEPATITIS TOXICA (ALCOHOL), DYSLIPIDEMIA - PURPLISH LIVER REFLECTION ZONE WITH A WHITE PEELING MEMBRANE

D. Hepatosplenomegaly

Fig. 99 The patient pictured below has had an enlarged liver and spleen for ten years, with increased transaminases, cholesterol, and uric acid, attributable to working with toxic construction materials. He has been diagnosed with pneumosclerosis, hypertonia, dyslipidemia, arrhythmia, gout, hyperthyroidism, hiatal hernia, and chronic gastritis. The liver and spleen reflection zones are swollen and are light pink to white in color. The liver reflection zone contains a dark brown spot (smaller arrow). The lower lip shows increased turgor.

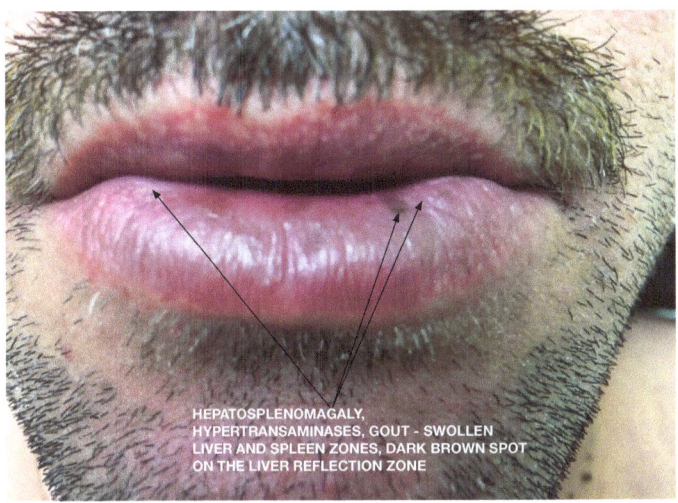

HEPATOSPLENOMAGALY, HYPERTRANSAMINASES, GOUT - SWOLLEN LIVER AND SPLEEN ZONES, DARK BROWN SPOT ON THE LIVER REFLECTION ZONE

Lip Diagnostics

Fig. 100 The patient below has diabetes mellitus, hepatosplenomagaly from working with heavy metals, increased transaminases and uric acid, hypertonia, arrhythmia, dyslipidemia, struma, and gastritis. The liver and spleen reflection zones are swollen and are light pink to reddish in color. The lower lip demonstrates increased turgor. The pancreatic reflection zone contains a red crack and a vertical line through the lower lip. A red crack can be seen on the stomach reflection zone, as well.

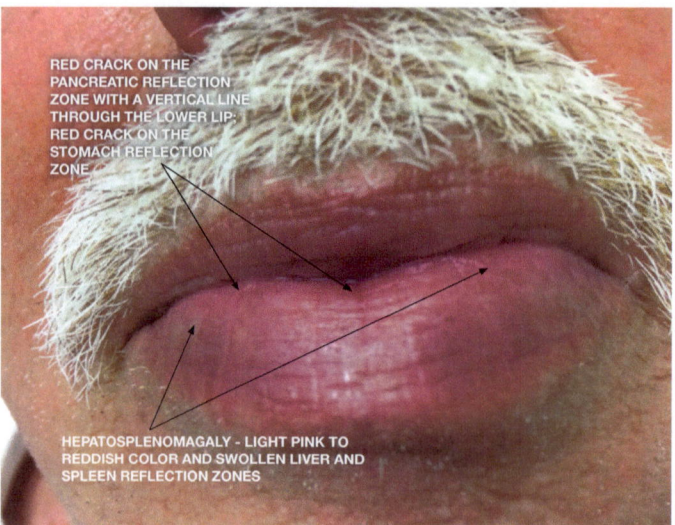

Fig. 101 The patient in the photograph below has an enlarged liver and spleen, chronic bronchitis, mitral valve prolapse, arrhythmia, and dyslipidemia. The liver and spleen reflection zones are swollen and light pink to purplish in color. The lower lip shows increased turgor.

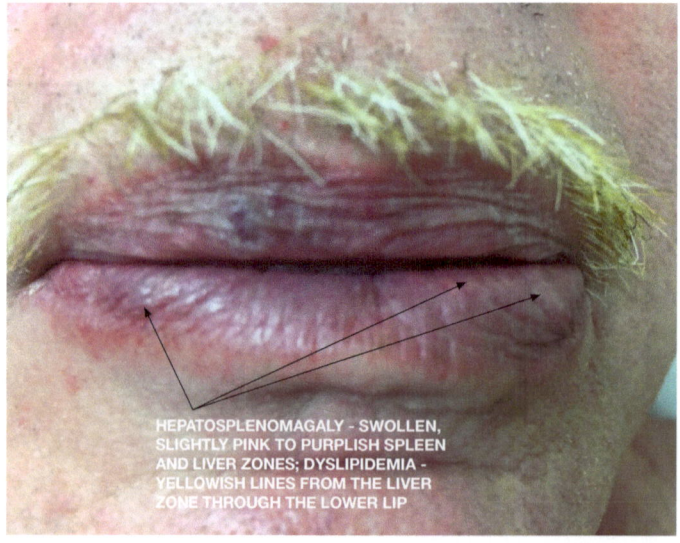

78 *Manifestations of the Diseases on the Lip Organ Zones*

Fig. 102 The patient pictured below has an enlarged liver, spleen, and pancreas. He smokes, and has overeaten sweet foods. The reflection zones of the liver, pancreas, and spleen are swollen and pink to reddish in color. The lower lip shows increased turgor.

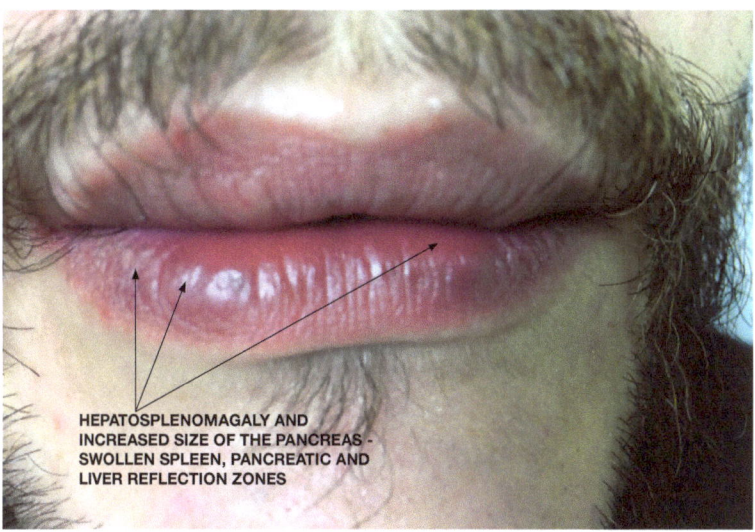

E. Hepatic Steatosis (Fatty liver). Dyslipidemia (Elevated cholesterol)

Fig. 103 The patient below has steatosis of the liver, dyslipidemia, and latent diabetes mellitus. The liver reflection zone contains light yellowish spots and a line at an angle across the lower lip (arrows).

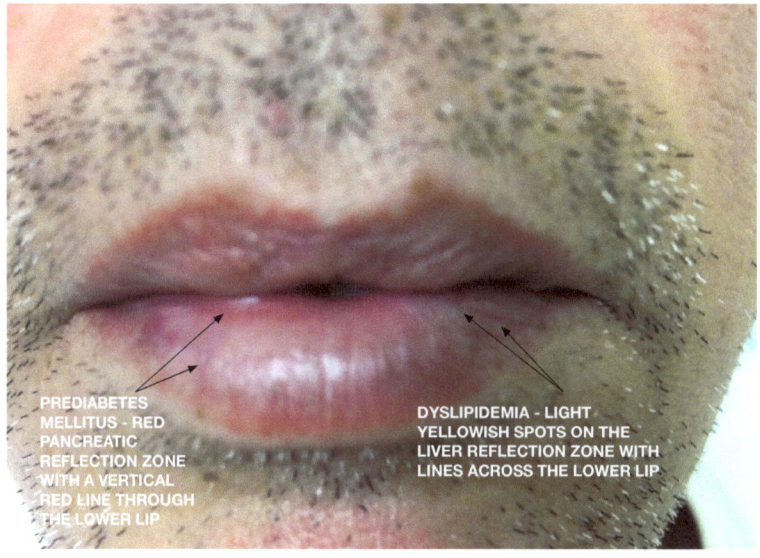

Fig. 104 The patient below has steatosis of the liver and dyslipidemia . Red vertical lines and light yellowish spots can be seen on the liver reflection zone (arrows).

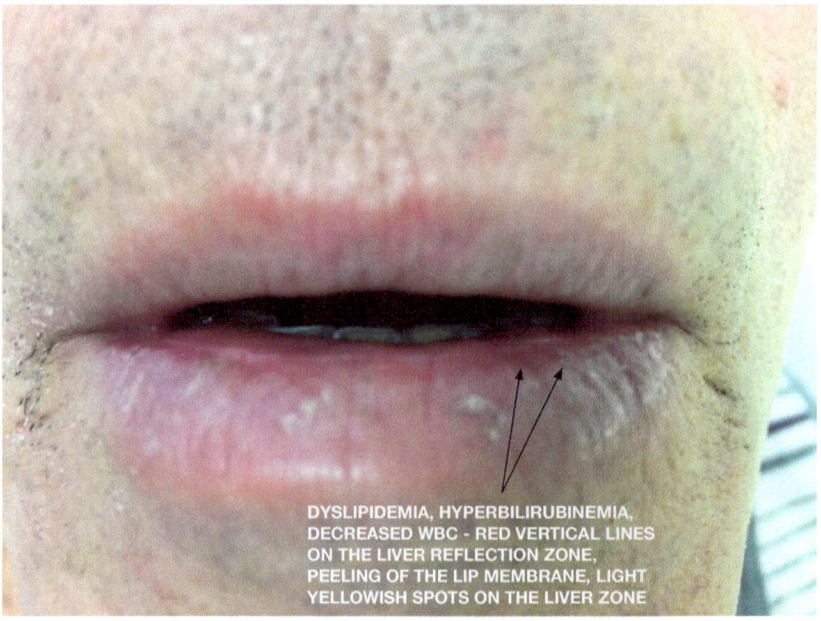

Fig. 105 The patient below with hepatic steatosis and dyslipidemia shows yellowish spots and a vertical crack on the liver reflection zone (arrows).

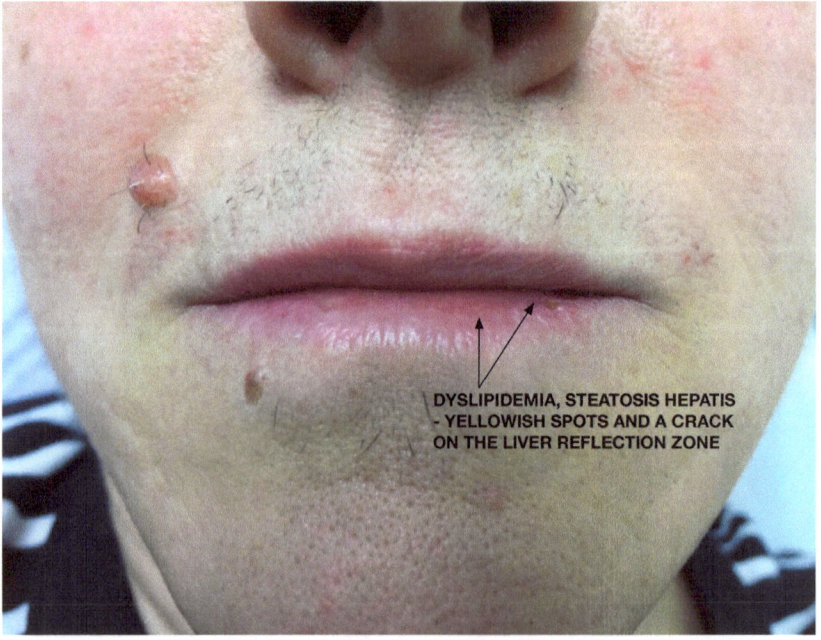

F. Hepatic cysts

Fig. 106 The patient below has multiple liver cysts. The liver reflection zone contains many vertical and angular folds (arrows). The liver reflection zone is slightly swollen.

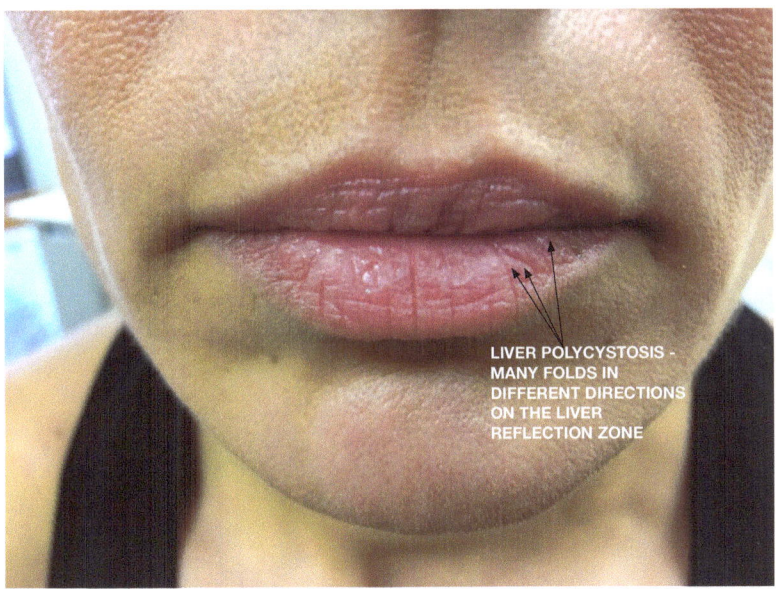

LIVER POLYCYSTOSIS - MANY FOLDS IN DIFFERENT DIRECTIONS ON THE LIVER REFLECTION ZONE

Fig. 107 The patient below has two parasitic liver cysts. The liver reflection zone contains two purplish bumps (arrows).

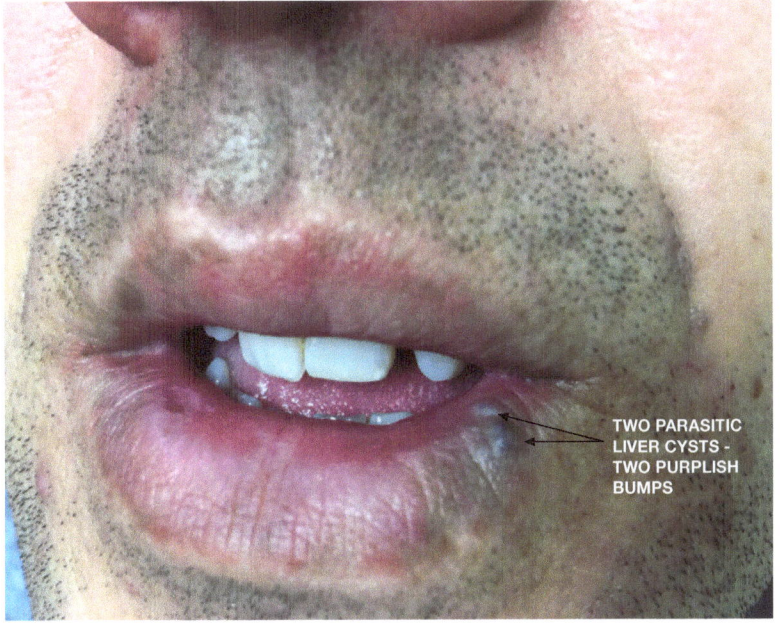

TWO PARASITIC LIVER CYSTS - TWO PURPLISH BUMPS

Fig. 108 The patient below has a liver tumor. The liver reflection zone contains a red spot (arrow). The membranes of the liver and stomach reflection zones are light pink in color and have a flat, polished surface.

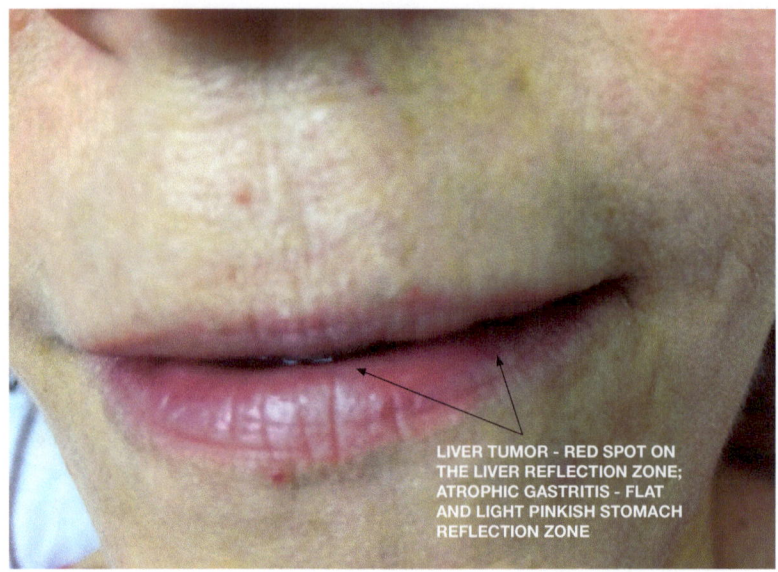

3.5. Cholecystitis. Cholelithiasis

Fig. 109 The patient below has gallstones and a chronic inflammation of the gall bladder characterized by pain, acid regurgitation, and abdominal distention.

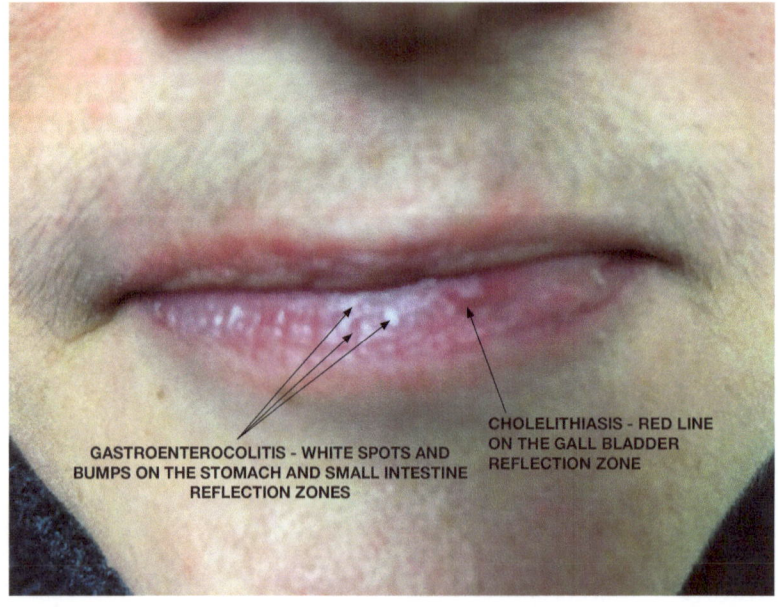

Fig. 110 The patient in the photograph below has two large gallstones. Two white bumps can be seen on the gall bladder reflection zone (arrows). Additionally, there are vertical red lines on the lower lip.

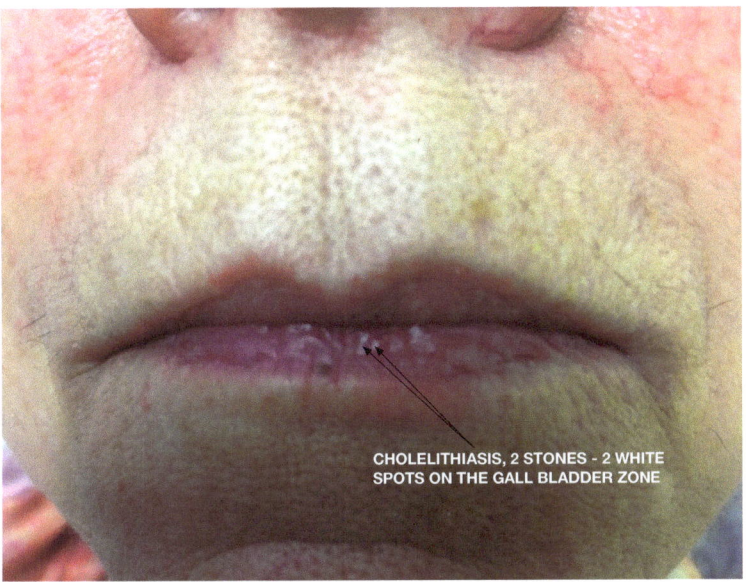

Fig. 111 The patient below has been diagnosed with cholelithiasis. The gall bladder reflection zone contains a transversal light pink to white line that spreads to the liver reflection zone on the right side and to the stomach and pancreatic reflection zones on the left side.

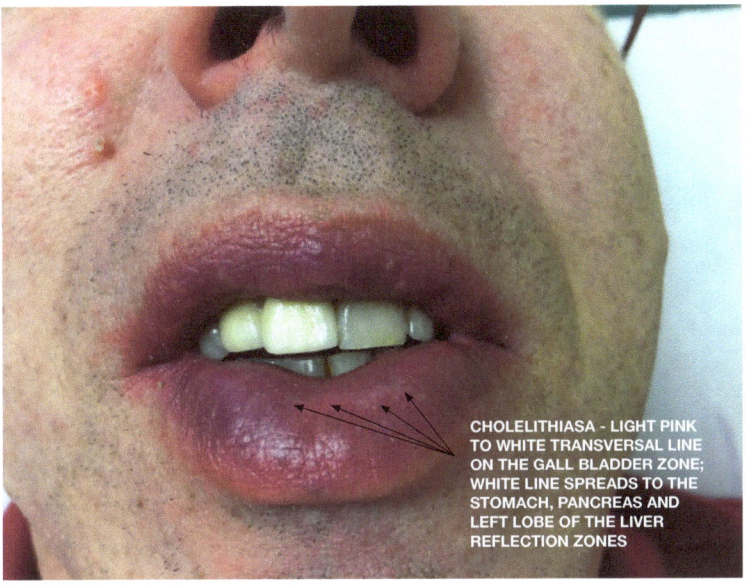

4. Pathologic Processes of the Urogenital System

4.1 Cystitis. Prostatitis

Fig. 112 The patient below has acute cystitis, a hypertrophic prostate, and pre-diabetes mellitus. The bladder and prostate reflection zones are dilated (marked by the black dots), and swollen. They contain an eroded red vertical line. The membrane line has spread from these zones to below the lower lip (arrow). The patient has pre-diabetes. Note the white, swollen spot on the pancreatic reflection zone.

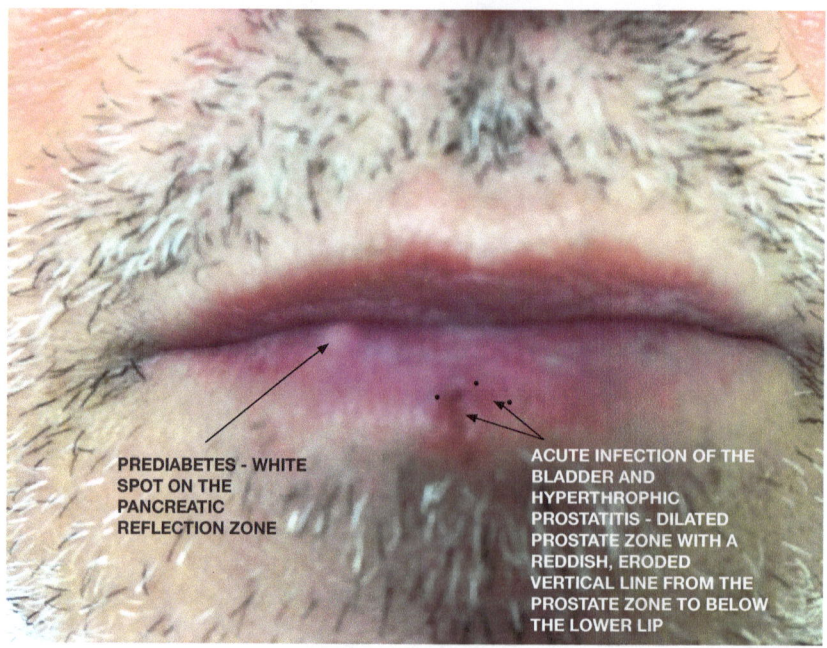

Fig. 113 The patient on next page has an acute infection of the bladder and prostate. The hypertrophied prostate is pressing and blocking the flow of urine in the urethra. The bladder and ureters are full of urine, resulting in hydronephrosis of the kidneys on the left side more than on the right side. The bladder and prostate reflection zones contain a brown spot. The left ureter and pylon reflection zones (hydronephrosis) contain a white line and a spot that marks the dilated zones.

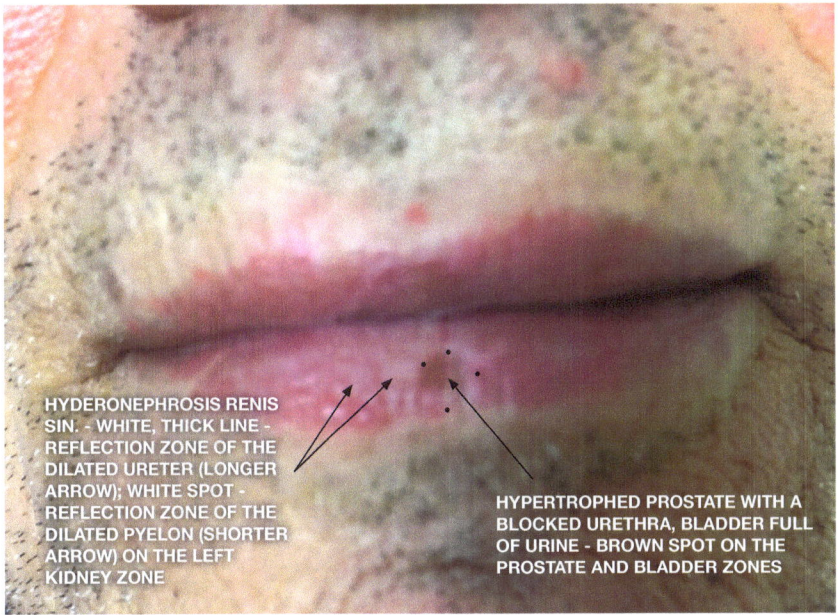

Fig. 114 The patient below has a chronic infection of the prostate and bladder that spread to the left kidney and caused a cyst to develop. The dark spot indicates chronic prostatitis and cystitis in the reflection zones. A white spot, representing the cyst, is seen on the left kidney reflection zone.

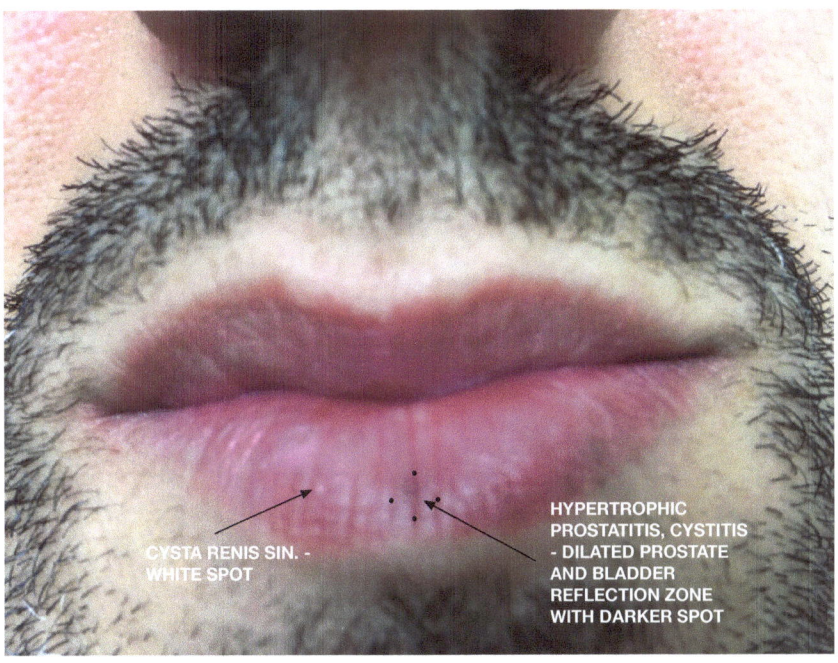

Fig. 115 The patient below has chronic cystitis, ptosis, and diverticulosis on the right side. The bladder reflection zone is light purplish pink, dilated (marked by the black points) and contains a red spot. The right side of the bladder reflection zone shows the diverticulosis. Note the darker spot.

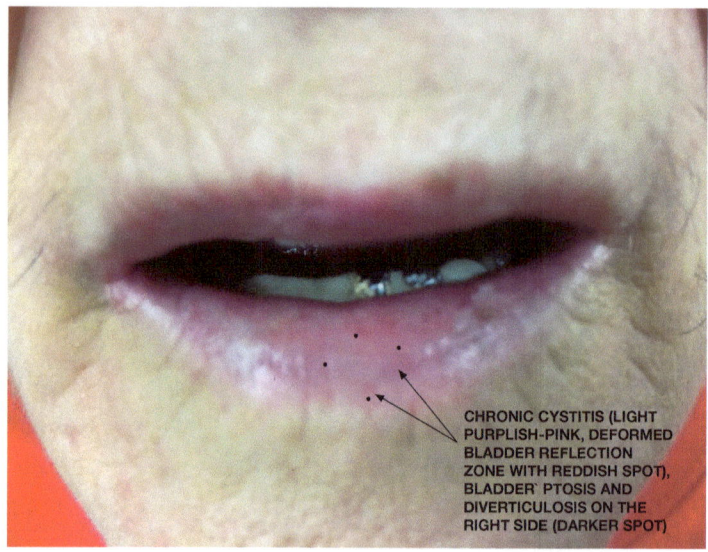

Fig. 116 The patient below has chronic prostatitis and cystitis. The prostate and the bladder reflection zones are dilated (marked by the black points), have a light pinkish purple color, and contain two transverse lines, indicating the replacement of glandular tissue with connective tissue.

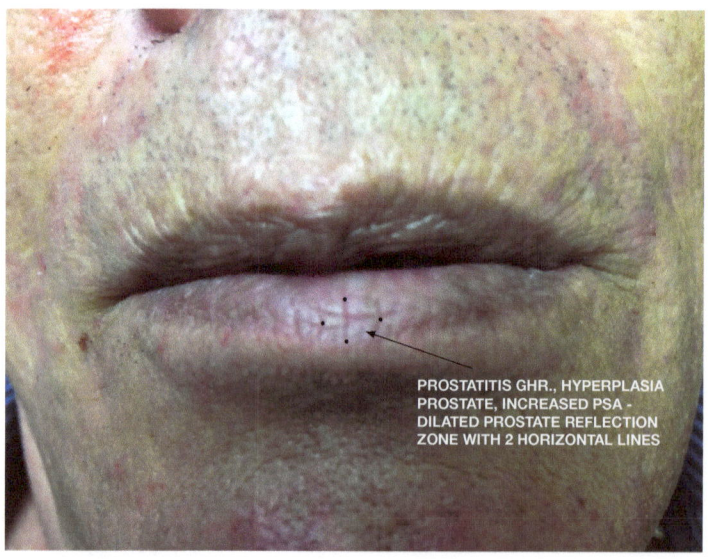

4.2 Glomerulonephritis. Kidney insufficiency

Fig. 117 The patient below has kidney insufficiency, increased creatinine, and a shrunken right kidney with a cyst measuring 2.8 x 2.6 cm. The right kidney reflection zone shows decreased turgor. The many small folds indicate a decrease in the size of the kidney (nephrosclerosis), and the purplish bump shows blood stasis, and a cyst. The left kidney reflection zone is slightly swollen and contains small purplish and white bumps indicating compensatory hyperplasia.

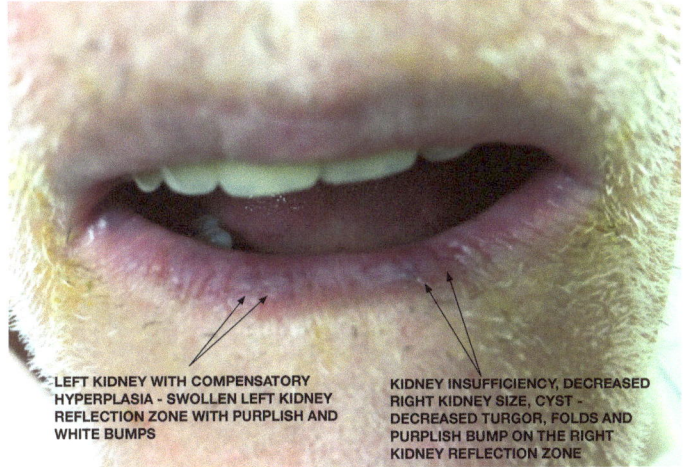

Fig. 118 The patient below has diabetic glomerulonephritis; kidney insufficiency characterized by an increase in creatinine and BUN (blood urea nitrogen); decreased GFR; anemia; and hypertonia. The kidney reflection zones are light pink and contain a transversal line signaling the replacement of functional tissue with connective tissue (nephrosclerosis).

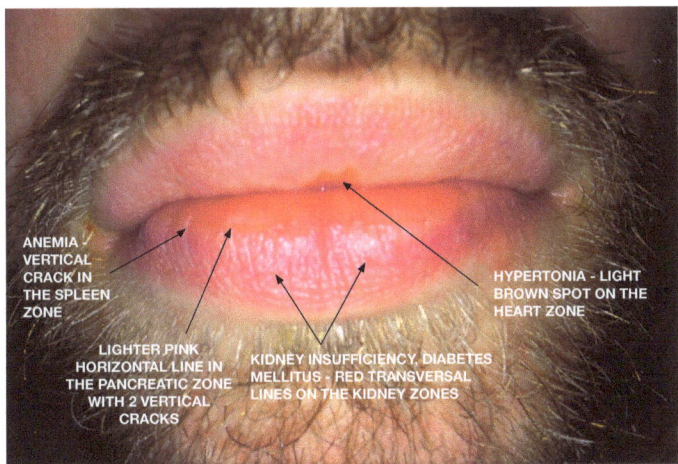

Lip Diagnostics

Fig. 119 The patient below has toxic glomerulonephritis and kidney insufficiency. The kidneys show a decrease in size (nephrosclerosis sin > dex). The kidney reflection zones contain transversal lines. The left kidney reflection zone displays a purplish bump representing the kidney with the most severe nephrosclerosis.

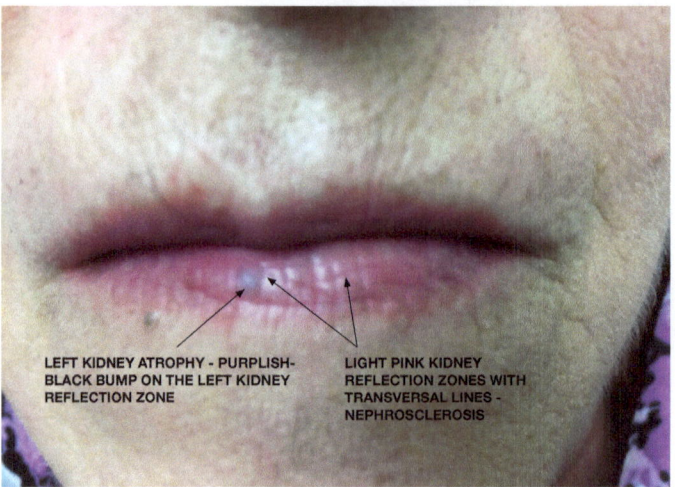

4.3 Nephrolithiasis

Fig. 120 The patient below has hydronephrosis which is more pronounced on the right side than the left, nephrolithiasis bilateralis, and hypertonia renalis. The kidney reflection zones contain brown spots. The brown spot on the right kidney reflection zone, indicative of the more pathologically changed kidney, continues as a brown vertical line to below the lower lip. The kidney reflection zones contain small dark spots indicating stone formations.

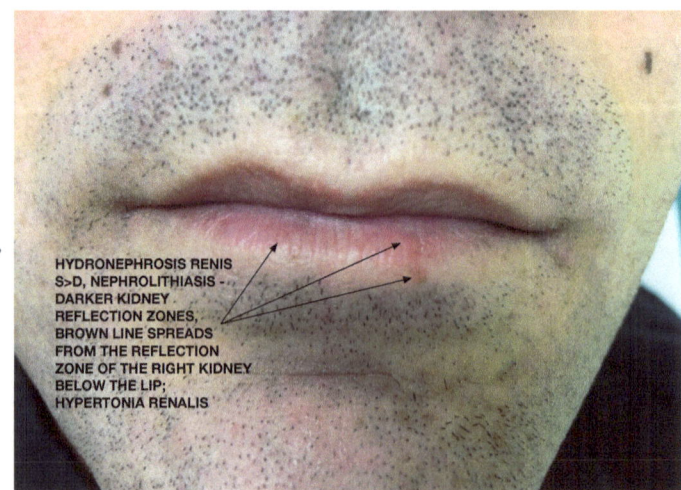

Fig. 121 The patient below has nephrolithiasis that is more advanced on the left side than the right. The reflection zones of the kidneys contain small dark points, representative of the stones. The left kidney reflection zone contains multiple small bumps expressing the manifestation of the stasis process.

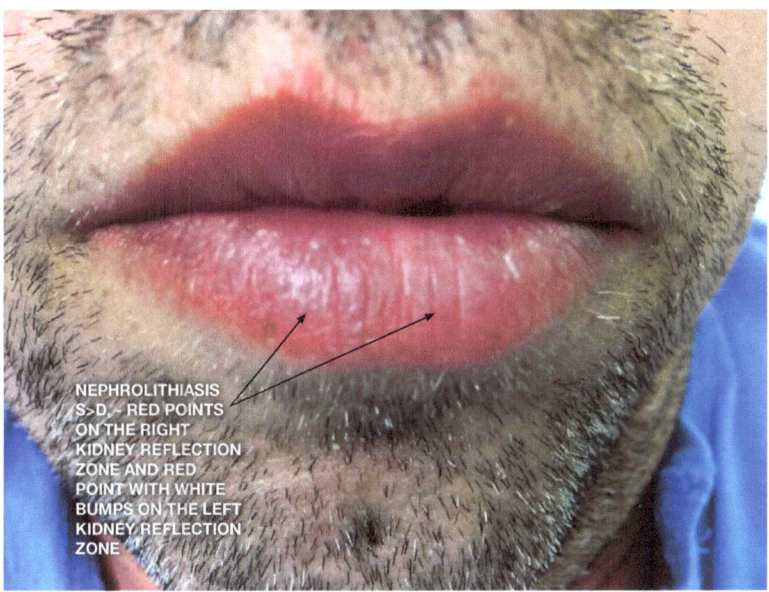

Fig. 122 The patient below has nephrolithiasis. The kidney reflection zones contain dark spots with red points.

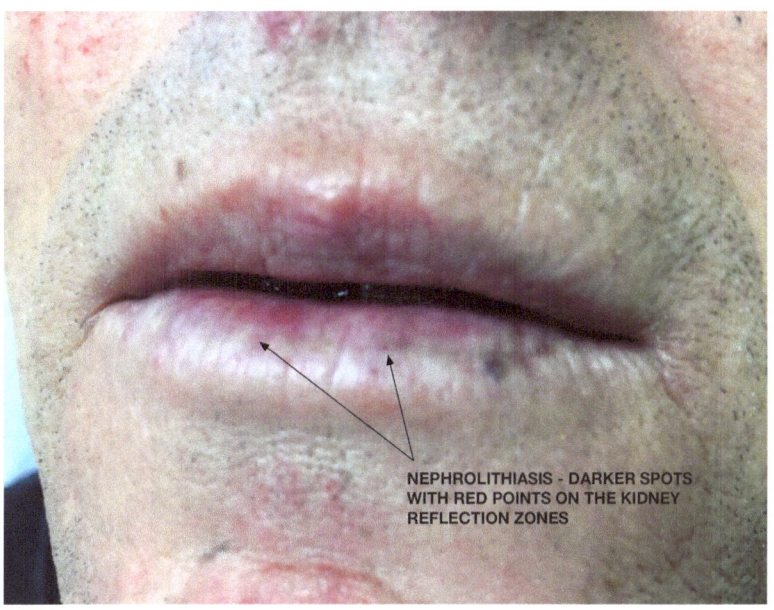

4.4 Tumors of the Urogenital System

Fig. 123 The patient below has a cyst on the left kidney. The left kidney reflection zone contains a brown spot (arrow).

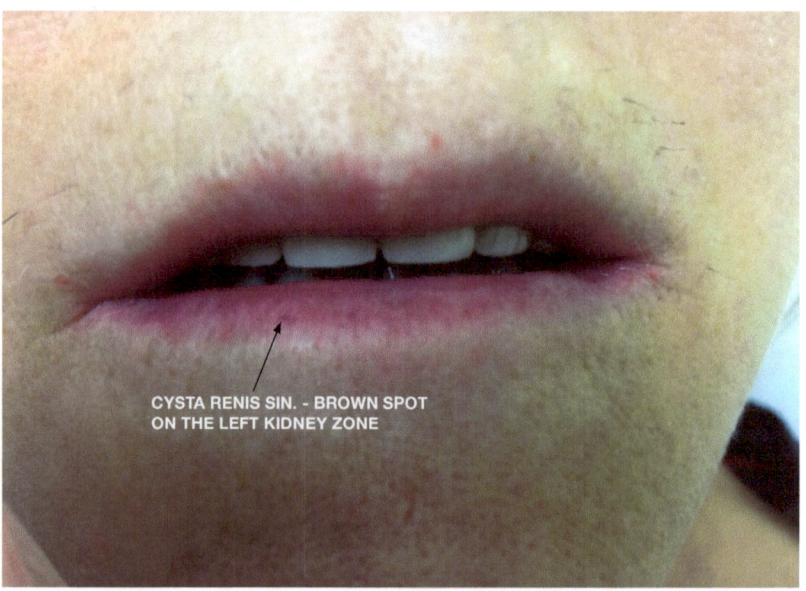

Fig. 124 The patient below has a cyst on the right kidney. The right kidney reflection zone contains a purplish spot (arrow).

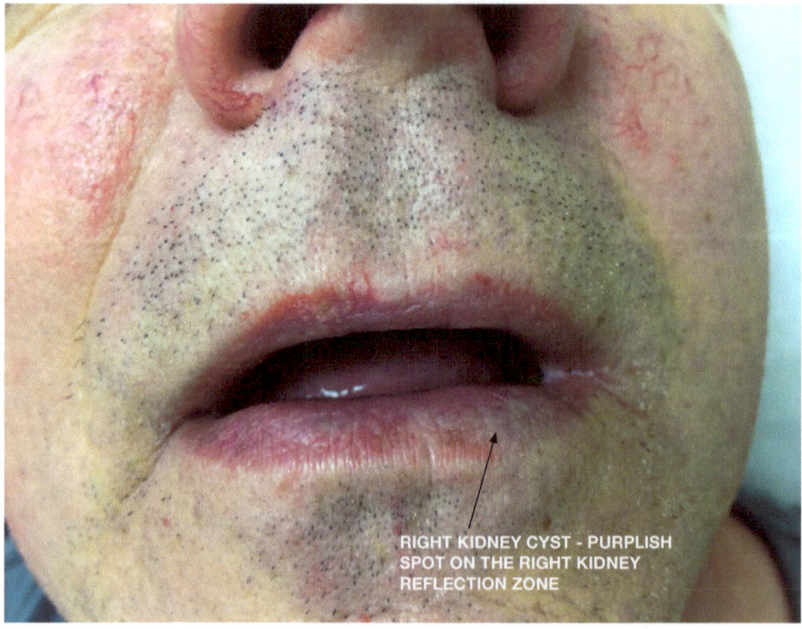

Fig. 125 The patient below had surgery on the right kidney because of a cancerous process and developed nephritis, a syndrome characterized by proteinuria and hematuria. The reflection zones of the kidneys are light pink to white in color. The reflection zone of the right kidney is swollen and dilated (marked by the black points). The left kidney reflection zone contains a transversal line.

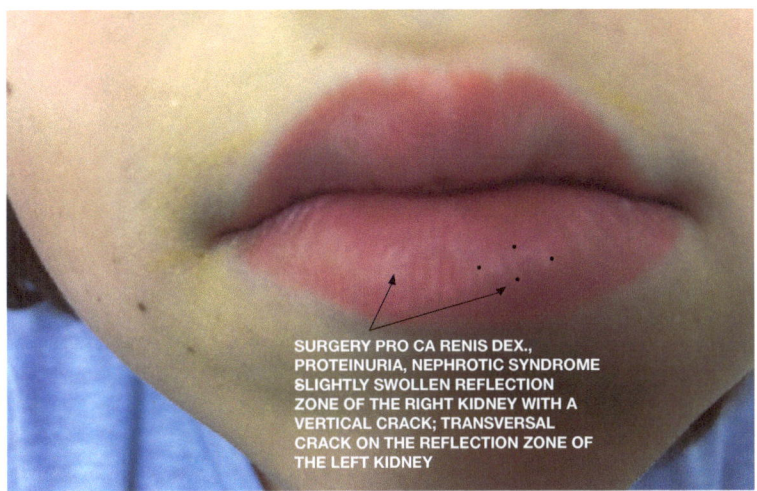

5. Pathologic Processes of the Endocrine System

5.1 Struma. Hyperthyroidism. Hypothyroidism

Fig. 126 The patient below has struma, hypothyroidism, and a cyst on the left thyroid lobe. The thyroid reflection zones contain red spots. The reflection zone pertaining to the left thyroid lobe has a big white bump, which indicates the cyst.

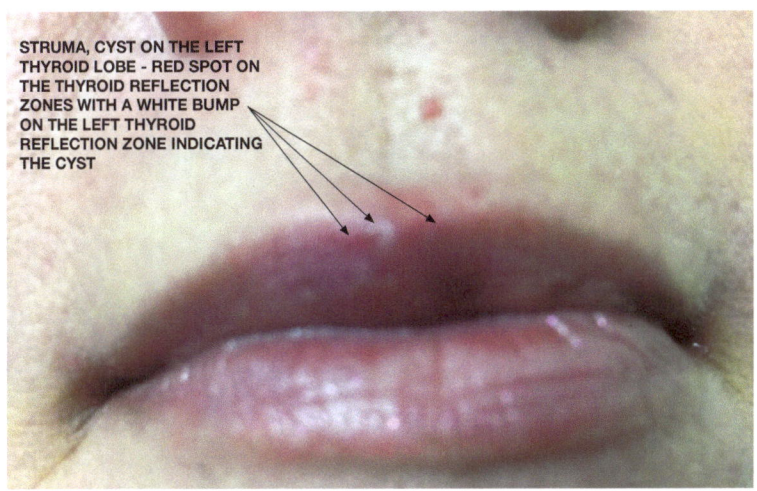

Fig. 127 The patient below has been diagnosed with struma and hypothyroidism. She was diagnosed with iodine insufficiency as a child but received iodine therapy. The thyroid reflection zones are reddish in color. A large bump formed above the left thyroid reflection zone in childhood.

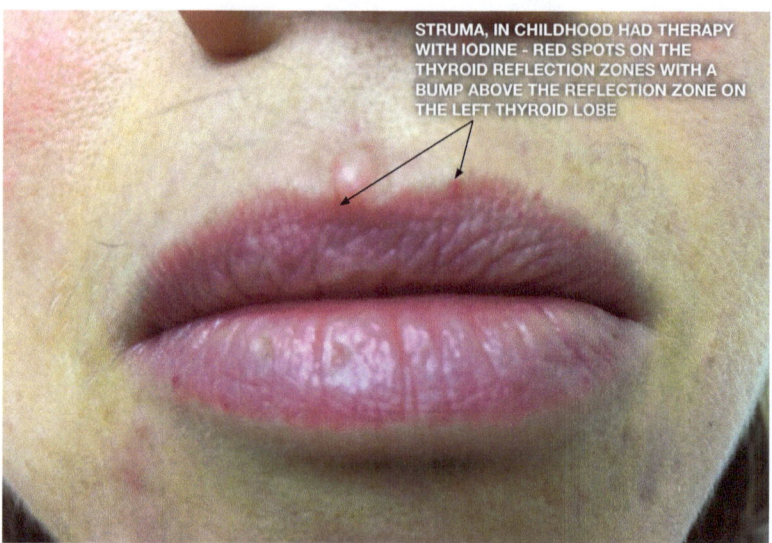

Fig. 128 The patient below has Hashimoto's thyroiditis, an autoimmune process of the thyroid gland, and hypothyroidism. The left thyroid reflection zone is slightly dilated and swollen, and is light pink. The right thyroid lobe contains a red point. The spleen reflection zone is swollen, a manifestation of the autoimmune process.

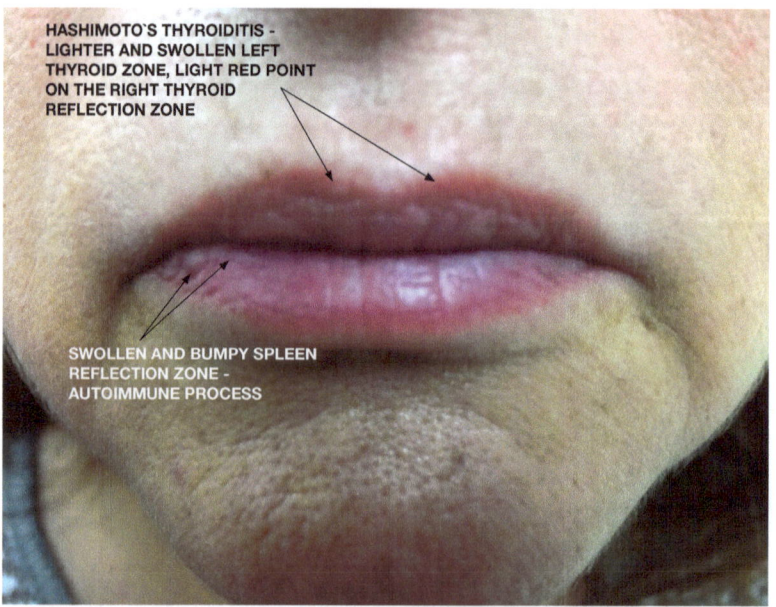

Fig. 129 The patient has a long history of Hashimoto`s thyroiditis and hypothyroidism. The left thyroid lobe reflection zone contained a brown spot that spread to above the lip membrane. The right thyroid reflection zone has been slightly replaced by skin, as a result of a long-term autoimmune process where glandular tissue was replaced by connective tissue. The spleen reflection zone is light pink and swollen, indicating an active autoimmune process.

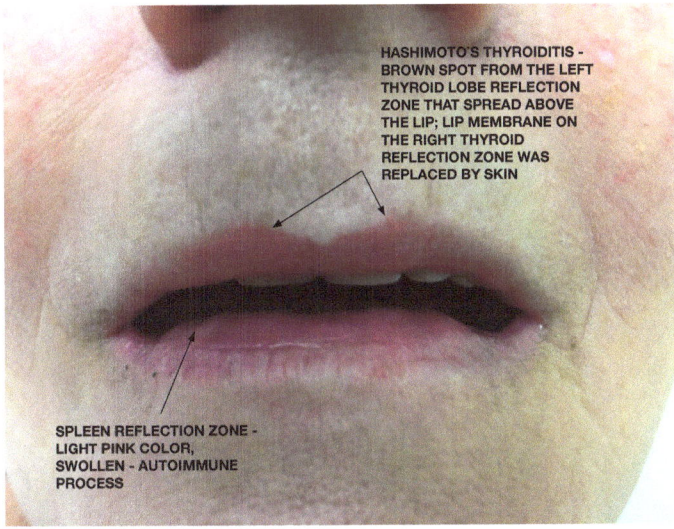

Fig. 130 The patient below has a long history of hypothyroidism. The lip membrane within the thyroid reflection zones has been partially replaced by skin. The left thyroid lobe reflection zone contains a small red point.

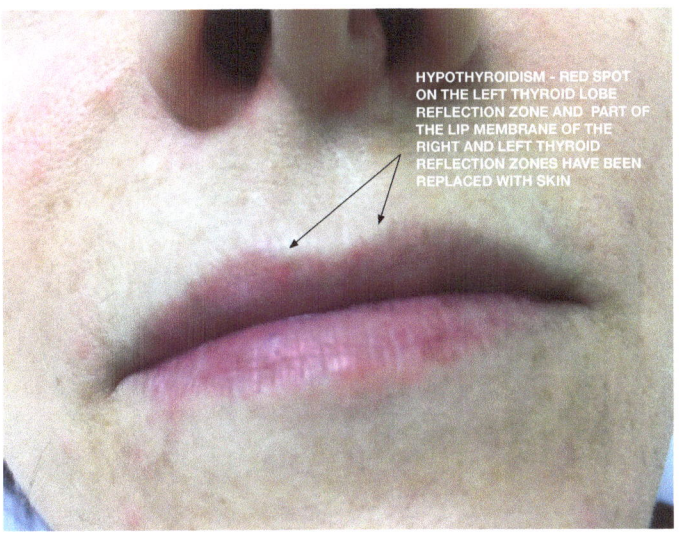

Lip Diagnostics

Fig. 131 The patient below has been diagnosed with hepatomegaly, struma, and the clinical symptoms of hyperthyroidism, such as sweating, palpitation, tremor, nervousness, and insomnia. His T3 and T4 levels are slightly elevated, and the TSH is below 0.5. Also, the patient is using stimulants. The thyroid reflection zones contain light pink to yellowish bumps. There are more bumps on the left thyroid lobe reflection zone than on the right. There is a light brown spot over the left thyroid reflection zone that spreads over the left brain reflection zone. Vertical lines start at the thyroid reflection zones. The vertical line beginning on the right thyroid reflection zone spread to the atrial reflection zone of the heart.

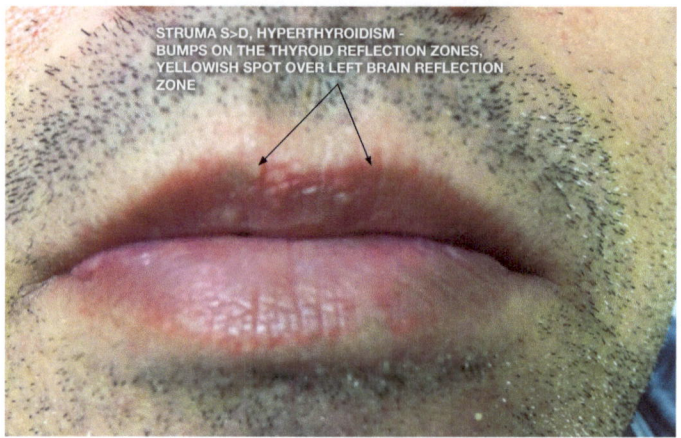

Fig. 132 The patient below has had hyperthyroidism since the age of eight, which was exacerbated by each pregnancy. The patient is experiencing palpitations, sweating, neurosis, and insomnia. The thyroid reflection zones are a light pinkish color and contain a tiny light yellowish bump. A brown line starting in the thyroid reflection zones stretches to above the lip membrane. The atrial reflection zone of the heart contains a similar light yellowish bump.

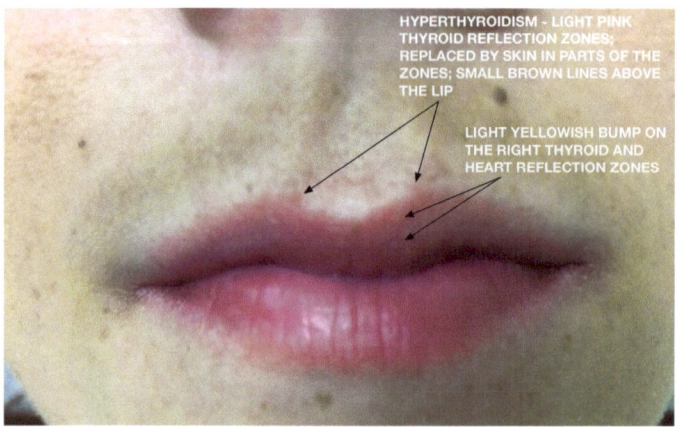

Fig. 133 The patient below has struma nodosa (goiter) and a cyst on the left thyroid lobe, although her thyroid hormone levels are normal. The left thyroid lobe area, reflecting the nodule and cyst, is dilated and exhibits light pink to white bumps. A vertical line starting at the bumps reaches to the heart reflection zone.

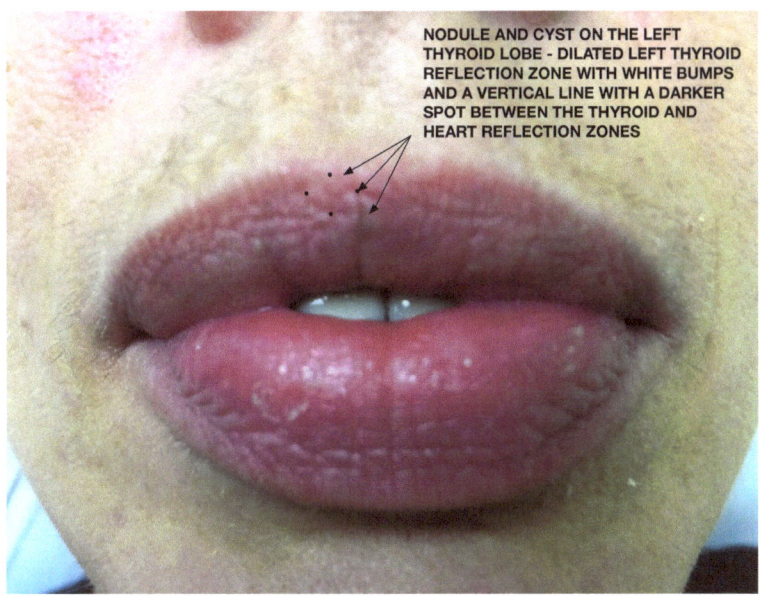

5.2 Diabetes mellitus

Patients with latent diabetes triggered by over eating sugary foods manifest a white spot with a vertical line in the pancreatic reflection zone on the lower lip. In a patient with developed diabetes mellitus (not enough insulin production) and with blood sugar over 120 mg%, the pancreatic reflection zone will be swollen, have a red or light pink color (when the condition is compensated with medication) and contain a white or darker vertical line in the lower lip. In cases of chronic diabetes, when the patient is on replacement therapy with insulin, the pancreatic reflection zone is flat, smooth (indicative of an atrophied pancreas), and is white or light pink in color.

Fig. 134 The patient below has latent diabetes, caused by an over consumption of sugary foods. The pancreatic reflection zone contains a white spot and a vertical line through the lower lip.

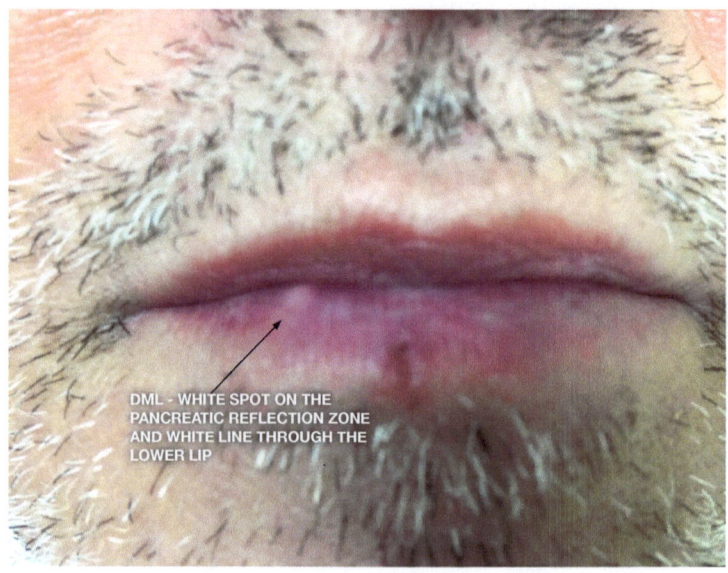

Fig. 135 The patient below, despite having a family predisposition to diabetes, consumes sugary food on a regular basis. Her blood sugar levels hover at around 120 mg%. The pancreatic reflection zone is red; the lip membrane is peeling and contains a light purplish spot.

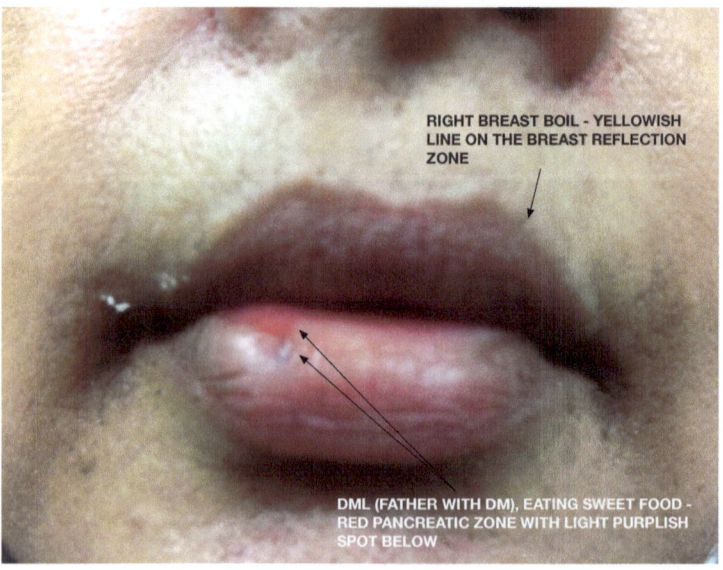

Fig. 136 The patient below has chronic diabetes mellitus, at a compensated stage, and is on Metformin. The pancreatic reflection zone is red to slightly brownish, the epidermis is peeling, and a white vertical line runs through the lower lip.

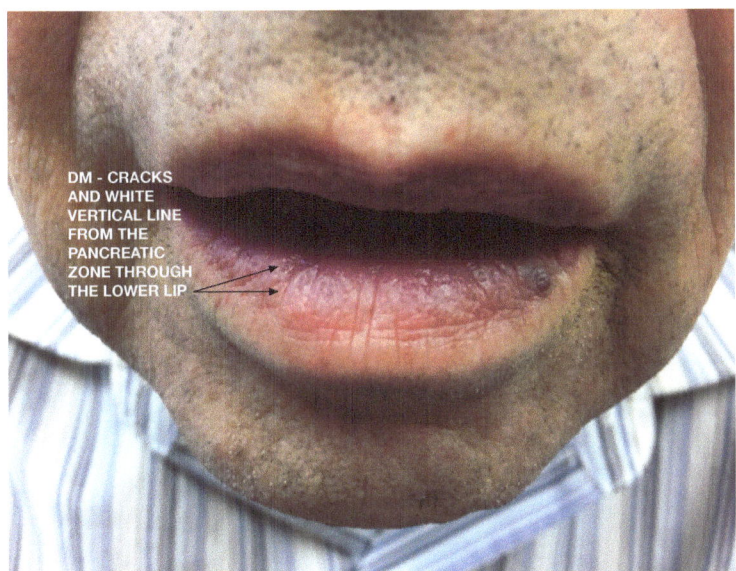

Fig. 137 The patient below has a long history of non- compensated diabetes. All of the reflection zones, including the pancreatic reflection zone on the lower lip are swollen and red in color. Two vertical lines have formed in the pancreatic reflection zone on the lower lip.

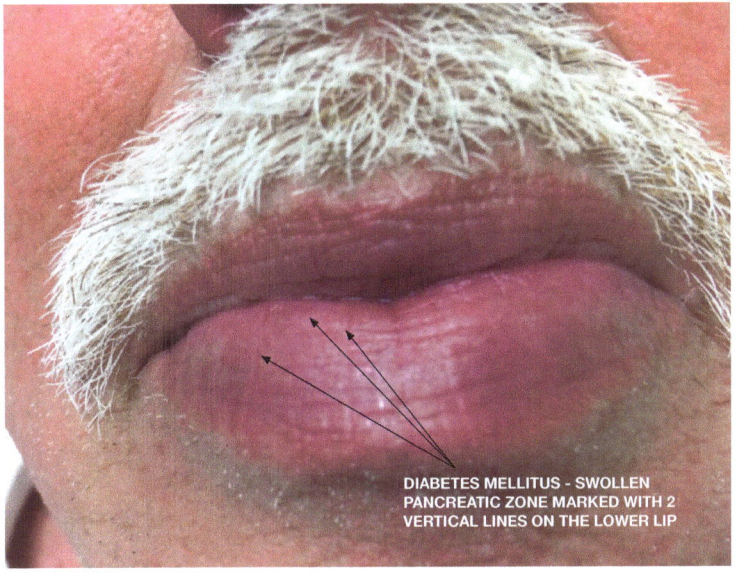

Lip Diagnostics

Fig. 138 The patient shown below has a long history of diabetes, unstable blood sugar levels, and is taking two anti-diabetic medications. The pancreatic reflection zone is swollen and light pink to white in color. A vertical line starting from a small red point in the pancreatic reflection zone crosses the lower lip. A second wide, white, vertical line is also seen on the pancreatic reflection zone of the lower lip.

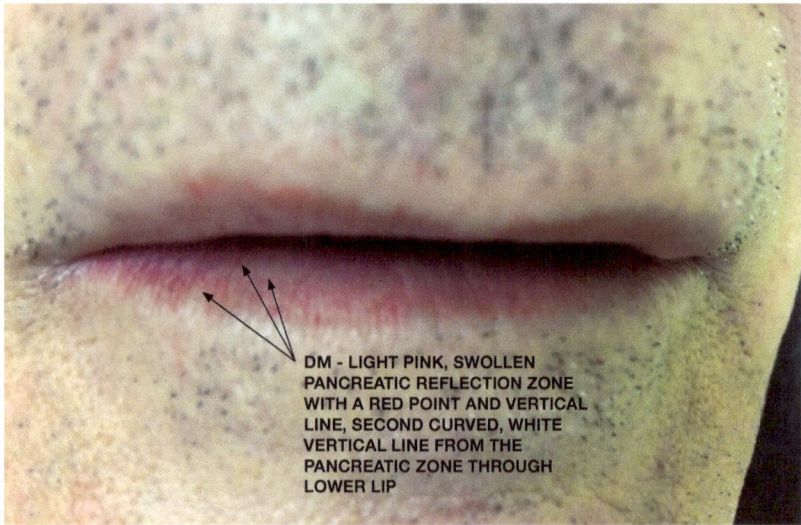

DM - LIGHT PINK, SWOLLEN PANCREATIC REFLECTION ZONE WITH A RED POINT AND VERTICAL LINE, SECOND CURVED, WHITE VERTICAL LINE FROM THE PANCREATIC ZONE THROUGH LOWER LIP

Fig. 139 The patient shown below has diabetes mellitus. The pancreatic reflection zone is light pink to white in color, contains a red point, and a vertical line that spans the height of the lower lip.

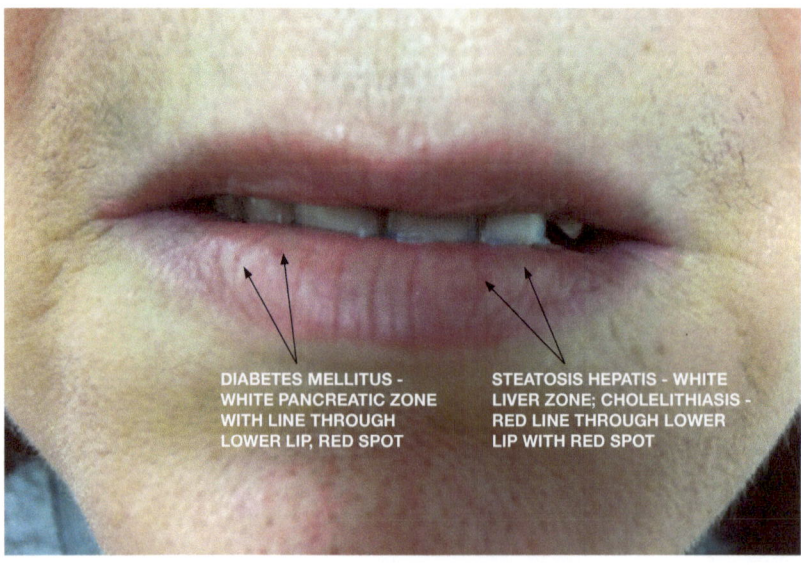

DIABETES MELLITUS - WHITE PANCREATIC ZONE WITH LINE THROUGH LOWER LIP, RED SPOT

STEATOSIS HEPATIS - WHITE LIVER ZONE; CHOLELITHIASIS - RED LINE THROUGH LOWER LIP WITH RED SPOT

Fig. 140 The patient shown below is exhibiting a light pink pancreatic reflection zone and a vertical white, wide line on the lower lip.

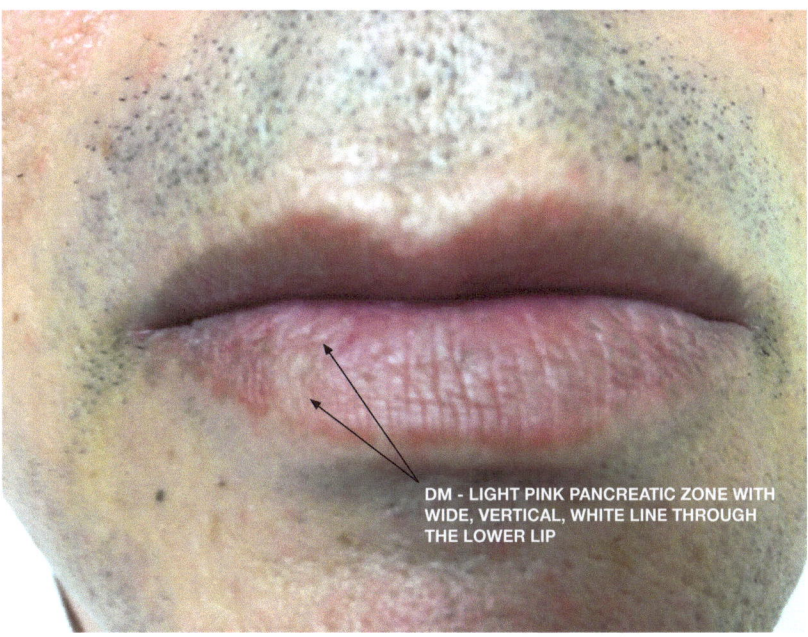

DM - LIGHT PINK PANCREATIC ZONE WITH WIDE, VERTICAL, WHITE LINE THROUGH THE LOWER LIP

Fig. 141 The diabetic patient below is exhibiting a pinkish red, swollen pancreatic reflection zone, and a white vertical line through the lower lip.

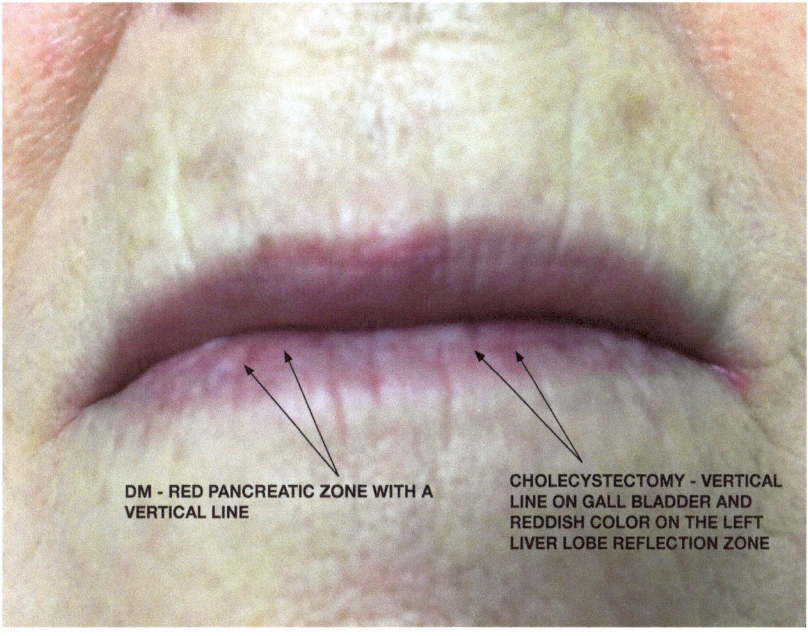

DM - RED PANCREATIC ZONE WITH A VERTICAL LINE

CHOLECYSTECTOMY - VERTICAL LINE ON GALL BLADDER AND REDDISH COLOR ON THE LEFT LIVER LOBE REFLECTION ZONE

Lip Diagnostics

Fig. 142 The patient below has a long history of diabetes mellitus. The pancreatic reflection zone is flat, reddish, and has a polished appearance. There is a dark vertical line running through the lower lip.

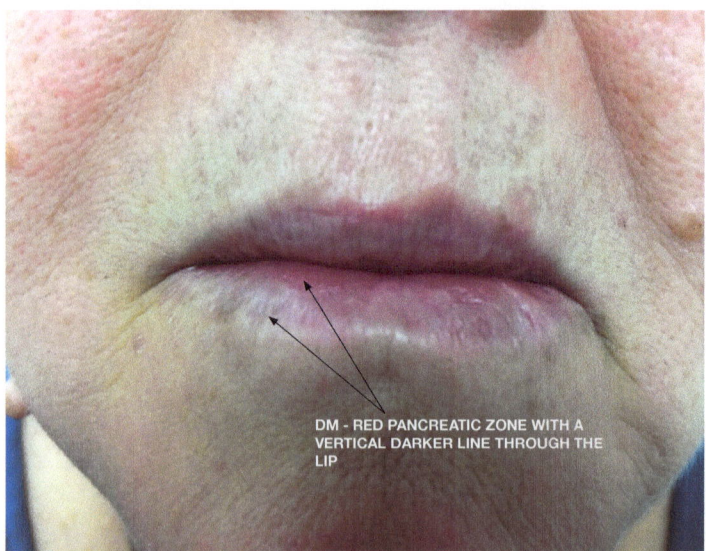

Fig. 143 The patient below has had diabetes mellitus for over twenty years. The patient exhibits side effects from diabetes, such as coronaro-angiopathy, glomerulo-nephropathy, retiono-angiopathy, and peripheral polyneuropathy. The pancreatic reflection zone is flat, light pink to white in color, contains a light reddish point, and a dark line through the lower lip.

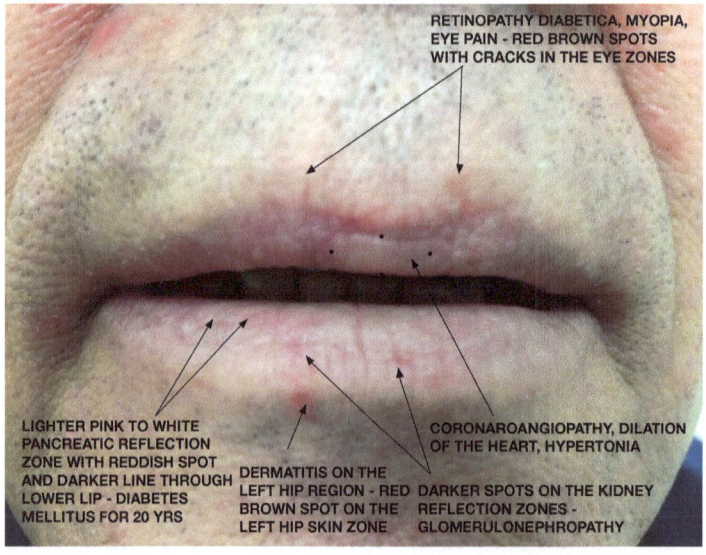

5.3 Infections and Tumors of the Uterus and Ovaries

Fig. 144 The patient below has acute ovarian and endometrial infections, a cyst on the right ovary (measuring 6.7x 5.0 cm), and small intramural uterine fibroma. Red, vertical lines have formed within the ovarian reflection zones of the lower lip (marked by the lateral arrows). A white spot, indicative of the cyst, can be seen on the right ovarian reflection zone (marked by the black points). There is a small, white bump on the uterine reflection zone indicating the fibroma (marked by the shortest arrow). The ovarian reflection zones are swollen and contain transversal folds that link to the uterine reflection zone.

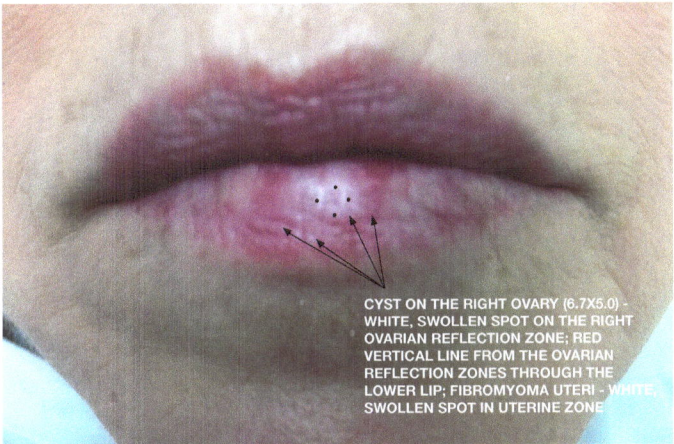

Fig. 145 The patient shown below has an endometrial infection, accompanied by vaginal discharge and pain. There is a fibroma on the left uterine horn and increased prolactin. The deep, red, vertical line through the uterine reflection zone of lower lip indicates endometritis, and vaginal discharge (longer arrow). The uterine reflection zone is reddish, and swollen. The reflection zone of the left horn contains a small white bump with a red point above it, indicating a fibroma (shorter arrow).

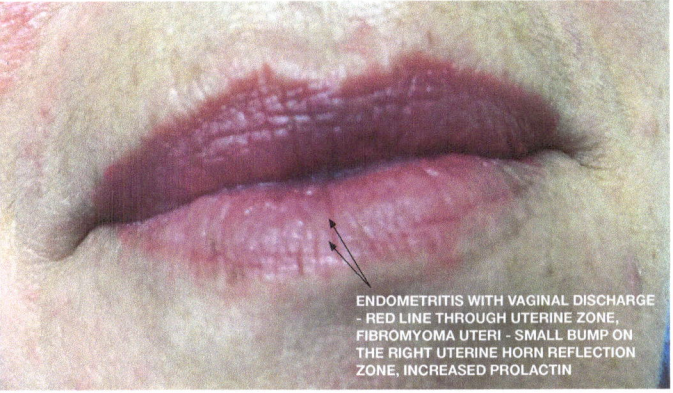

Lip Diagnostics

Fig. 146 The patient shown below has been bleeding from the uterus for three months (metrorrhagia), and has microcystosis of the ovaries. There is a vertical line (indicated by the arrow) through the uterine reflection zone. The uterine refection zone is swollen and bigger than the rest of the lip (marked by the black points). Very small dark dots can be seen on the ovary reflection zones.

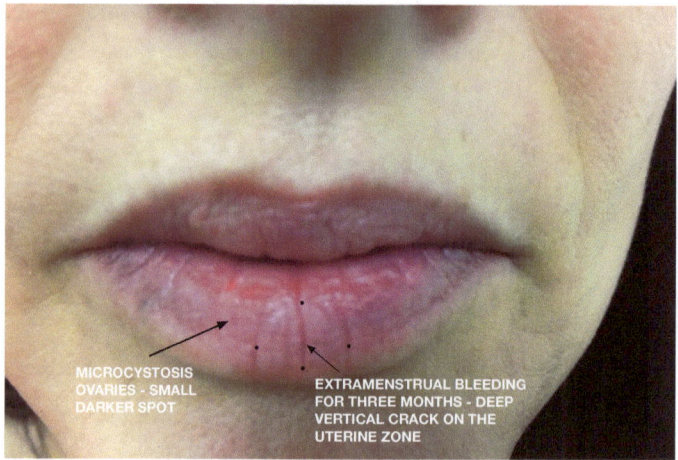

Fig. 147 The patient below was photographed after an ablation of the uterus for extra heavy menstrual bleeding. The uterus is enlarged, contains a fibromyoma, and there is a cyst on the right ovary. The uterine reflection zone is light pink to white in color. Note the white spot below the lip border. The red, swollen spot on the left side of the uterine reflection zone is indicative of the fibromyoma. The right ovarian reflection zone contains a white bumpy spot that has spread below the lip border, and is indicative of the cyst.

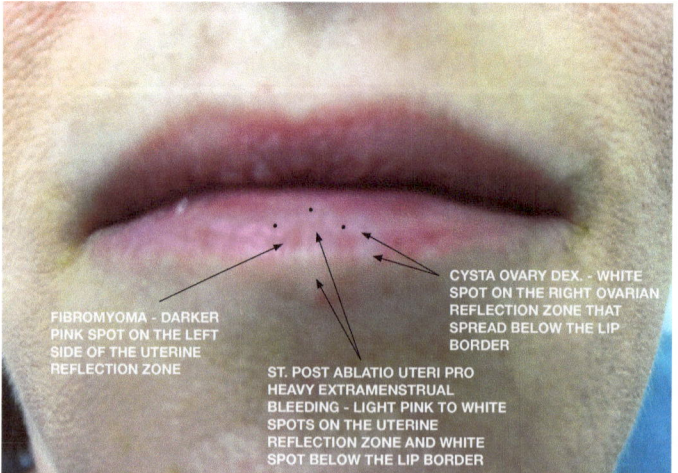

Fig. 148 The patient shown below has chronic endometritis characterized by pain and burning in the uterus. The uterine and left ovary reflection zones contain purplish bumps.

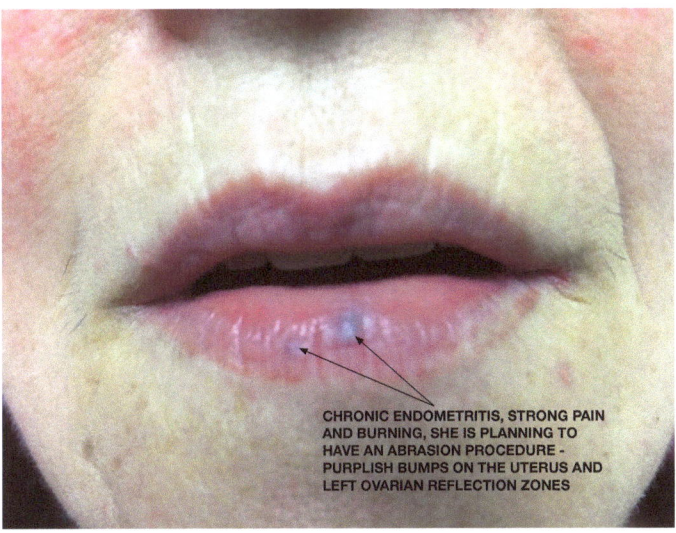

CHRONIC ENDOMETRITIS, STRONG PAIN AND BURNING, SHE IS PLANNING TO HAVE AN ABRASION PROCEDURE - PURPLISH BUMPS ON THE UTERUS AND LEFT OVARIAN REFLECTION ZONES

4.5 Tumors of the Genital System

Fig. 148 The patient shown below has a fibromyoma, or a benign tumor of the uterus. The uterus is enlarged, and the fibroma is localized within the left part of the uterus. The reflection zone of the uterus (marked by the black points) is swollen and light pink to white in color. The uterine reflection zone has a deformation on the left side (arrow).

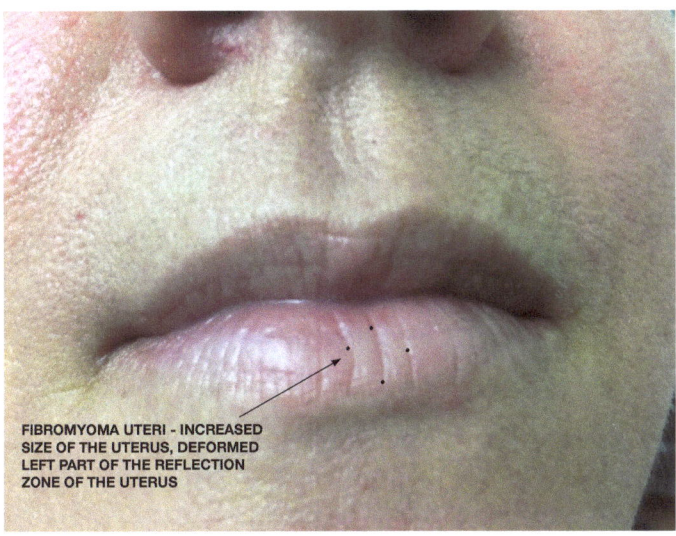

FIBROMYOMA UTERI - INCREASED SIZE OF THE UTERUS, DEFORMED LEFT PART OF THE REFLECTION ZONE OF THE UTERUS

Fig. 149 The patient shown below has an enlarged uterus (16.0x7.0 cm) with a large fibromyoma on the left side of the uterine fundus. The reflection zone of the uterus is enlarged (marked by black points) and light pink to white in color. The reflection zone of the left fundus contains a brown spot indicative of the fibromyoma (arrow).

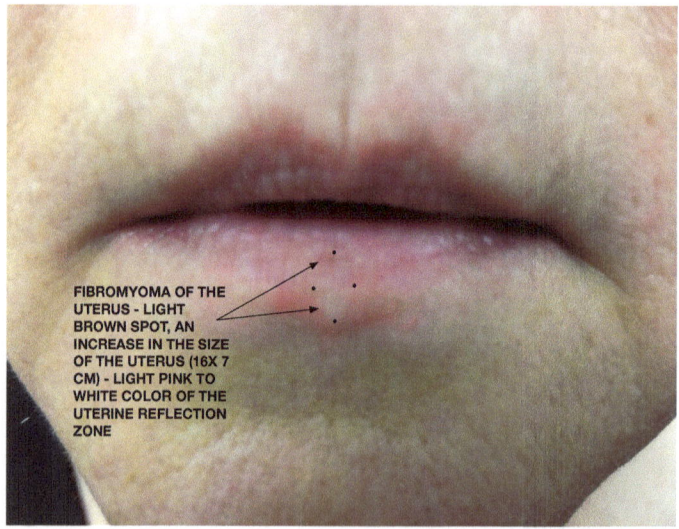

Fig. 150 The patient below had two abortions and has two very small fibromyomas. Two angular cracks, indicative of the abortions, along with two small white bumps (fibromyomas) on the fundal section of the uterine reflection zone can be seen (marked by the black points).

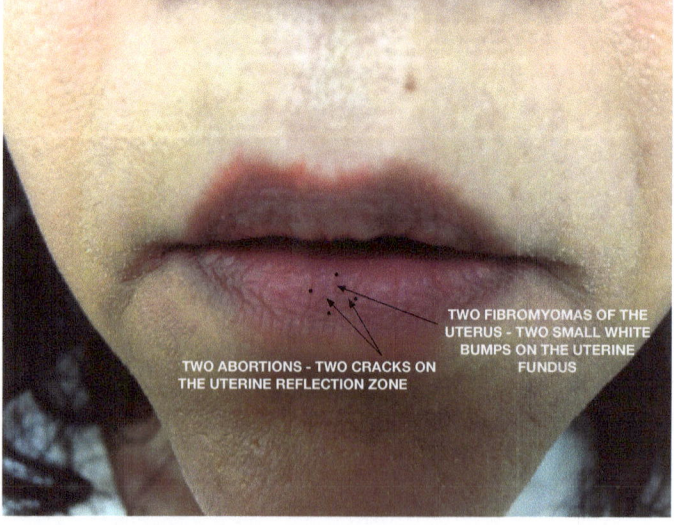

Fig. 151 The patient below has an enlarged uterus. The right side of the uterus has doubled in size and is bigger than the left side. A fibromyoma is growing out of the right uterine horn. The reflection zone of the uterus (marked by the black points) is enlarged and the right side has doubled in size. The reflection zone of the right horn contains a white spot that is indicative of the fibromyoma (arrow).

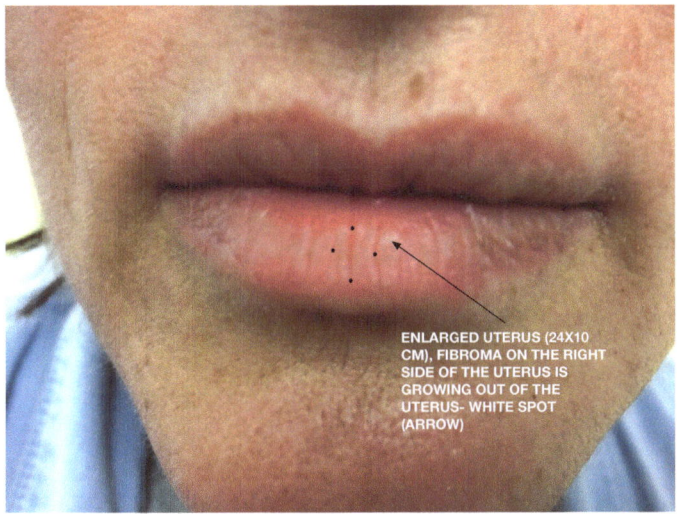

Fig. 152 The patient below is in menopause and has a painful cyst on the left ovary. The uterine reflection zone is light pink in color and contains a vertical line (marked by the black points). The left ovarian reflection zone contains a small white bump indicating a cyst (longer arrow). There is a red spot below the lip border that connects, through a fold, to the ovarian reflection zone. This is indicative of a chronic and painful cyst (shorter arrow).

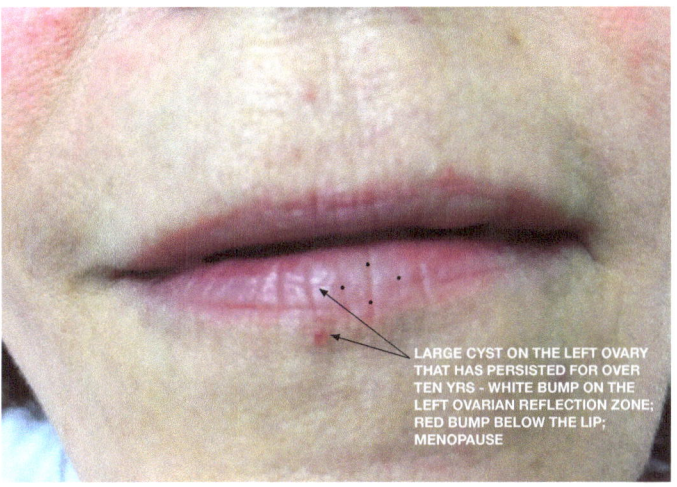

Lip Diagnostics

Fig. 153 The patient shown below had a total hysterectomy thirty years ago. The reflection zone of the uterus has decreased in size (marked by the black points).

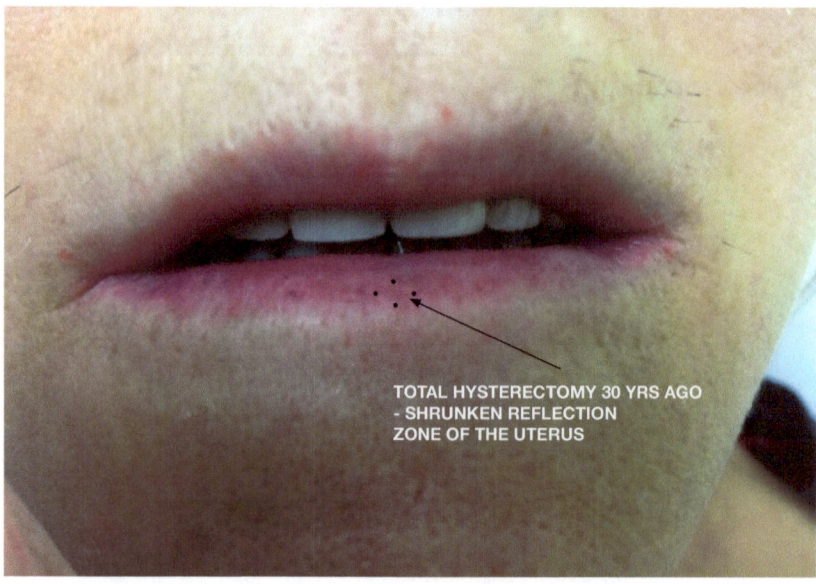

5.4 Breast

Fig. 154 The patient below has had a fibroma of the left breast for seven years. The left breast reflection zone contains a white vertical line that spread to above the upper lip border (arrow).

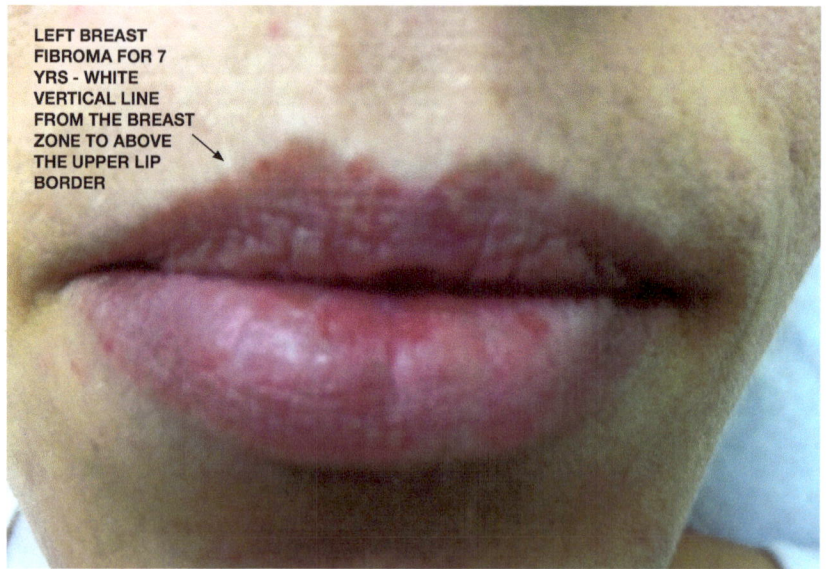

Fig. 155 The patient below has fibrocystosis of both the left and right breasts. The breast reflection zones are light yellowish in color and contain red points.

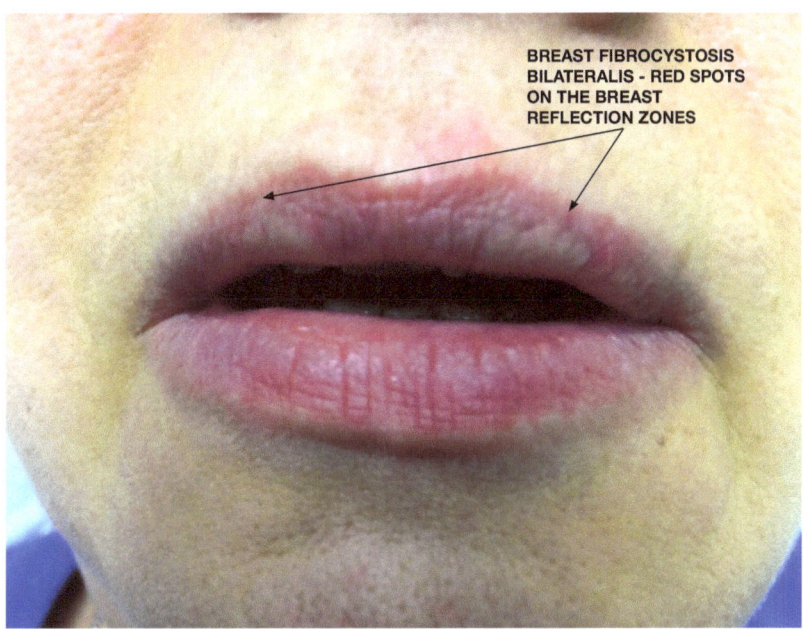

Fig. 156 The patient below had surgery thirty years ago for polycystosis of the breasts. The cysts were more prevalent on the right side of the body than on the left side. The breast reflection zones contain brown spots (arrows).

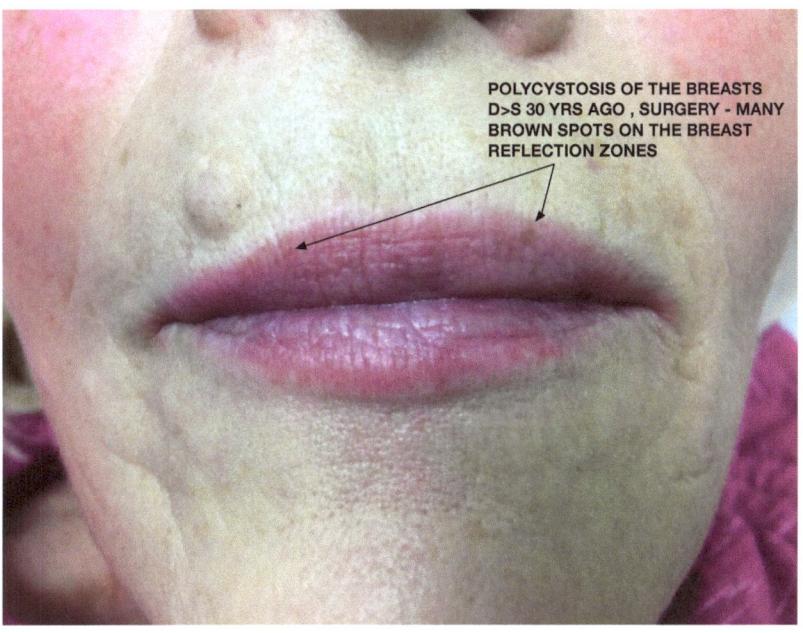

Lip Diagnostics

Fig. 157 The patient below had cancer of the right breast - two cancerous nodules. The right breast reflection zone contains two red spots (arrows). A vertical yellowish line starting at the second, deeper red spot crosses the breast reflection zone.

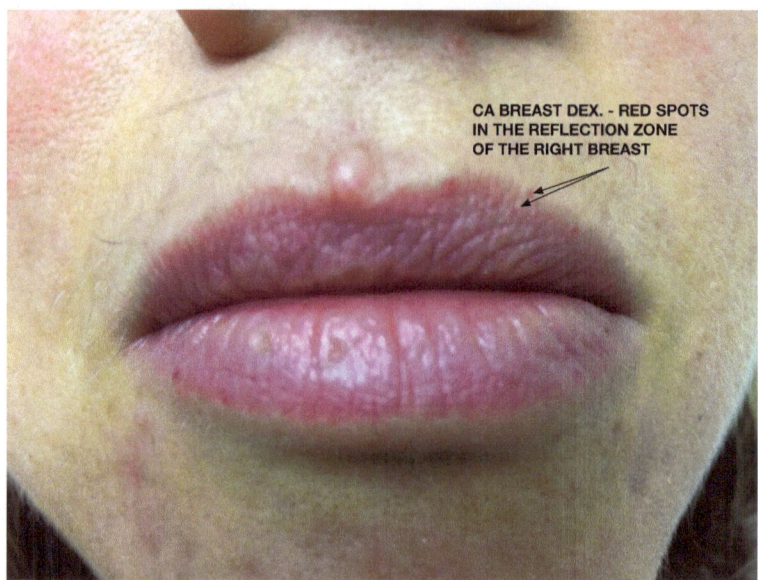

Fig. 158 The patient below has a boil on the right breast. She has latent diabetes from overeating sugary foods. The right breast reflection zone contains a yellowish vertical line.

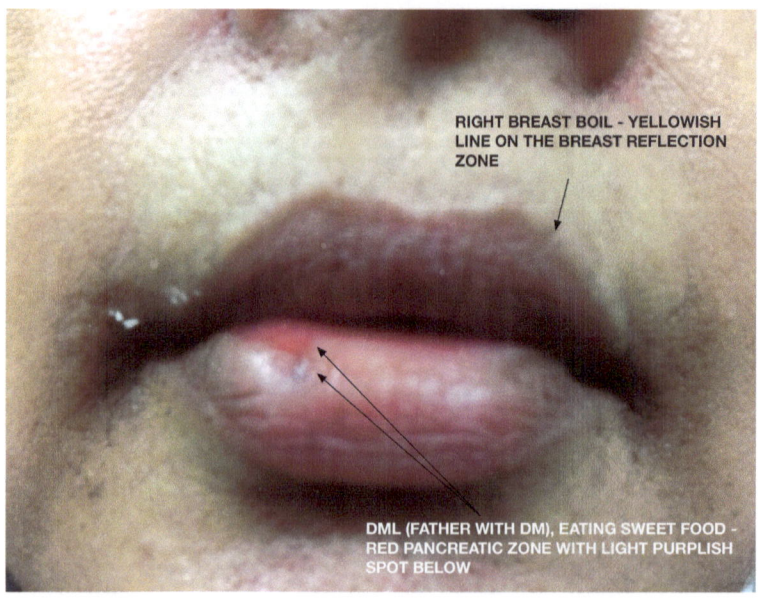

108   *Manifestations of the Diseases on the Lip Organ Zones*

Fig. 159 The patient below has been diagnosed with fibrocystosis of the breasts that are more prevalent on the left side. The breast reflection zones contain brown points, which are more visible on the left side than on the right side (arrows).

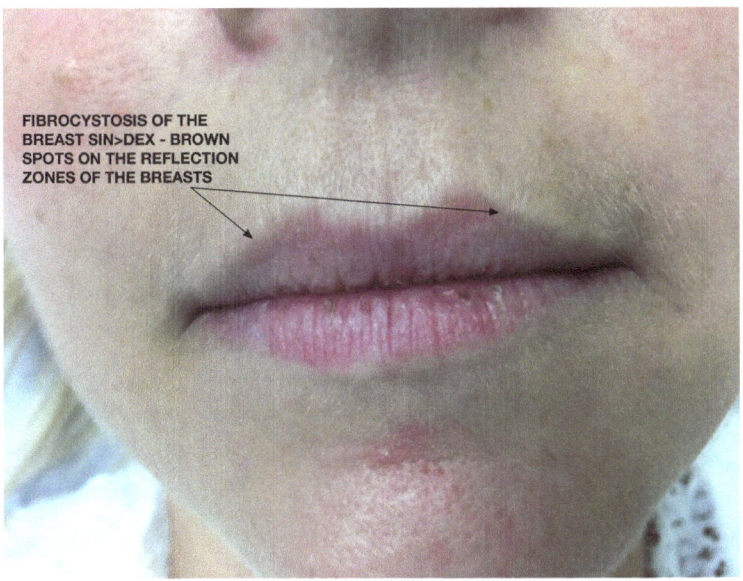

6. Pathologic Processes of the Brain and Peripheral Nervous System

6.1 Neuroses

In most cases, patients with anxiety, panic attacks, and neuroses, accompanied by palpitations, shortness of breath, sweating, tremors, disturbed sleep, impatience, and fear have an overactive thyroid gland and hypertrophy of the right thyroid lobe. The representation of anxiety, panic attack, and neurosis on the lips includes a white line over the upper lip border, a slightly dilated right thyroid lobe reflection zone with a vertical line to the atrial reflection zone of the heart (indicative of palpitations and sweating), dilated and swollen heart and lung reflection zones (indicating palpitations and hyperventilation), and a red or dark spot on the brain reflection zone.

Lip Diagnostics

Fig. 160 The patient below has anxiety, panic attacks, and obsessive-compulsive disorder. There is a white line over the upper lip. The right thyroid reflection zone is slightly dilated and contains vertical lines from both the right and left thyroid reflection zones to the heart reflection zone. The heart (marked by the black points) and the lung reflection zones are swollen, reddish, and dilated. The right brain reflection zone contains a dark spot.

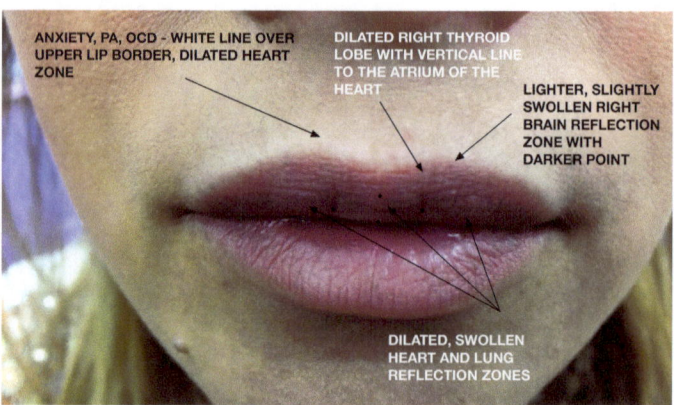

Fig. 161 The patient below has obsessive-compulsive disorder, anxiety, insomnia, and a struma. The lips are red and swollen. The thyroid reflection zones are dilated and contain a white, angular line from the right thyroid lobe and vertical lines from the left thyroid lobe to the heart reflection zone. The lung and heart reflection zones (marked by the black points) are dilated. The right brain reflection zone is darker in color. A lighter yellowish to white line is found above the upper lip border (not clearly visible because of the patient's moustache).

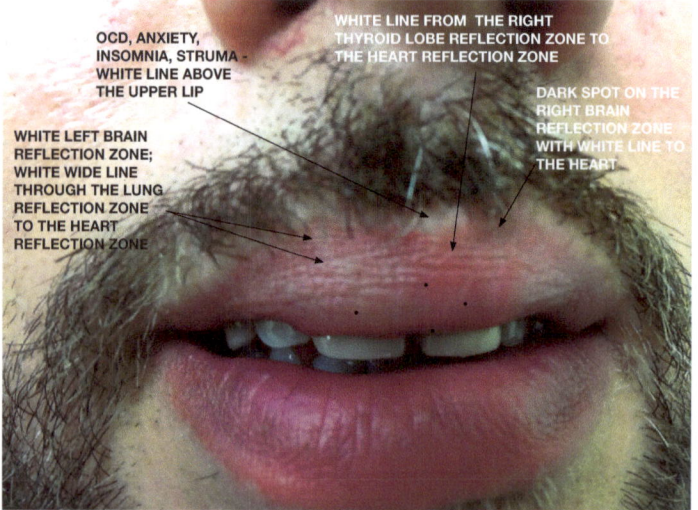

6.2 Headache. Migraine

Fig. 162 The patient shown below had a trauma to the right side of the nose. He periodically experiences headaches that start in the nasal area and spread to the eyes and forehead. There is a reddish brown spot on the right side of the nose reflection zone. Very tiny red, transversal lines start at the nose reflection zone and spread to the eye and forehead reflection zones. They are more visible on the left reflection zones.

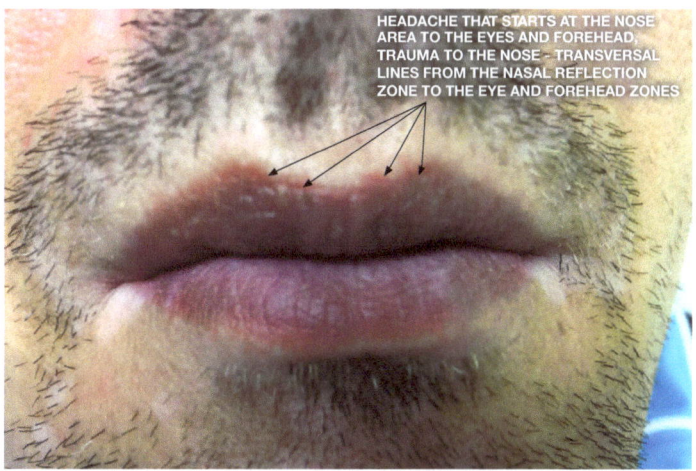

Fig. 163 The patient below has frequent headaches from eye strain. He is a (taxi, bus, truck) driver, whose headaches begin in the eye region and spread to the occipital region of the head and to the neck. The eye and brain reflection zones contain reddish brown spots that have spread to the neck reflection zones. There are wide, vertical, reddish lines above the eye reflection zones indicating that his eyes have been overtaxed for a long time.

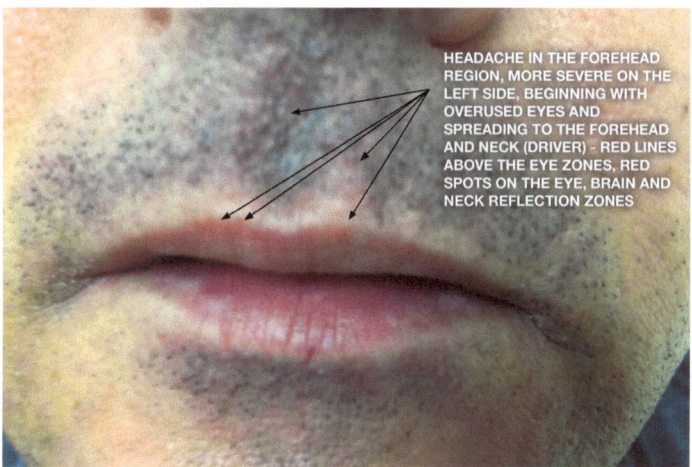

6.3 Tremors

It impossible to distinguish the type of tremor a patient has by using lip diagnostics only. There is only one sign of tremors that manifests on the lips – the formation of small, yellowish bumps on the zones reflecting the affected parts of the body. When therapy is effective, the number and size of the bumps decreases or disappears.

Fig. 164 The patient below has an essential tremor of the pectoral muscles and arms. His father had the same tremor. The lip reflection zones of the pectoral muscles and arms contain small yellowish bumps (indicated by the arrows).

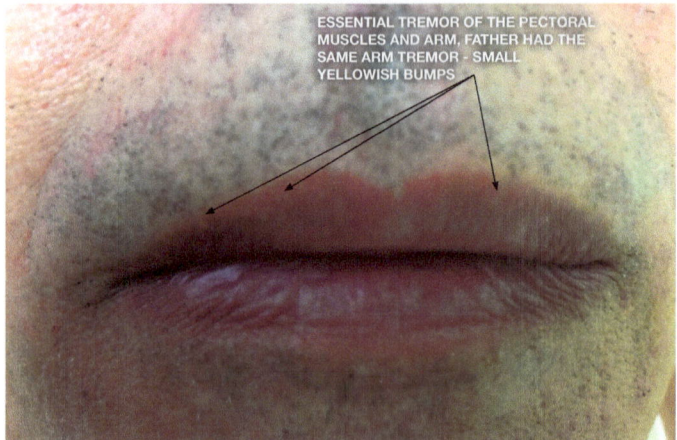

Fig. 165 The patient below has a tremor due to Parkinson's disease that manifests more on the left side of the body than the right. There are multiple small, yellowish bumps on the left arm and leg reflection zones (arrows).

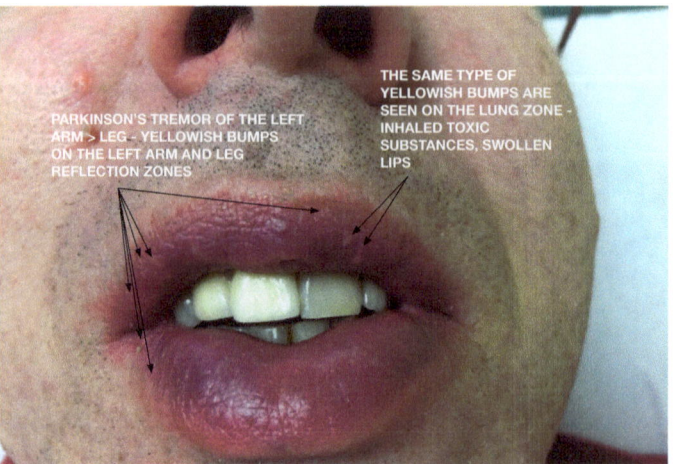

6.4 Paralyses

Fig. 166 The patient pictured below has developed anesthesia induced encephalopathy during knee replacement surgery. He has quadriparalyses (weakness in all four limbs), motor aphasia, hepato-splenomegaly, diabetes mellitus, and stenocardia. The brain reflection zones contain dark spots and lines from the throat and lung reflection zones to the brain reflection zone, due to the toxic influence of the anesthesia. The reflection zones of the most affected extremities (right arm and left leg) are lighter pink to yellow in color and are narrowed. There are deep folds at the corners of the mouth. A vertical line can be seen in the right knee reflection zone, signaling the knee replacement.

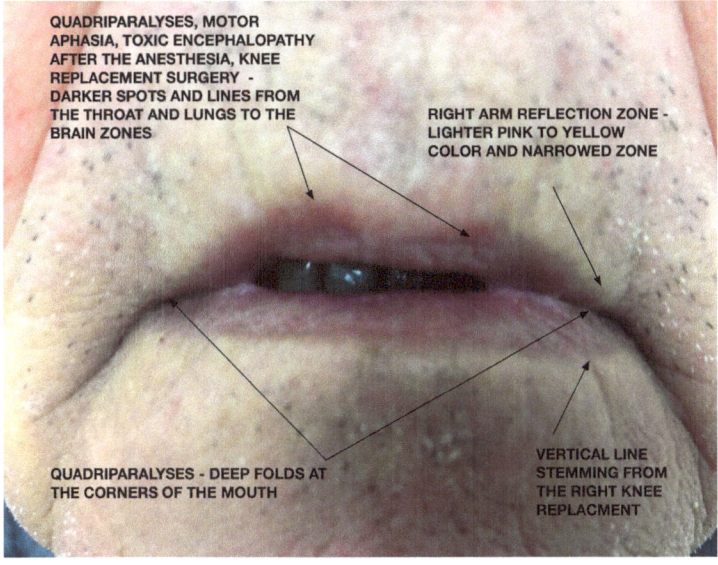

Lip Diagnostics

Fig. 167 The patient shown below has post-traumatic quadriparalyses that has had a greater impact on the right arm and the legs. There is a yellowish line on the spine, right arm, and leg reflection zones. The right arm and leg reflection zones are slightly narrowed.

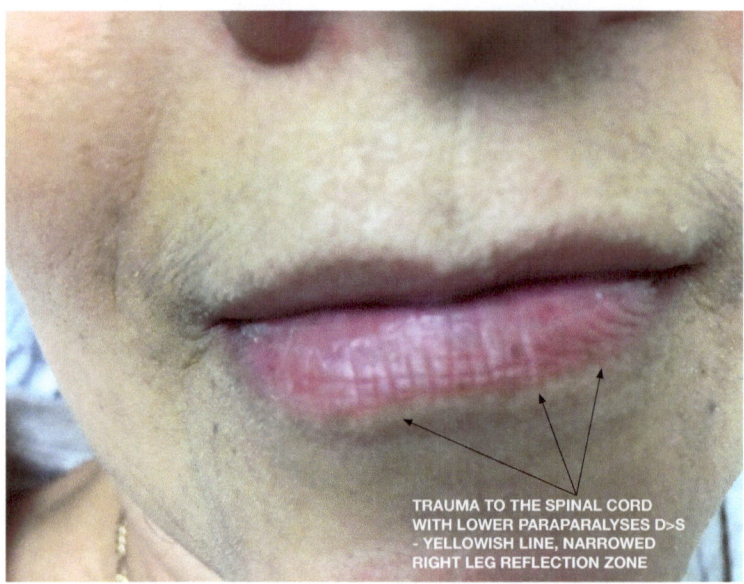

TRAUMA TO THE SPINAL CORD WITH LOWER PARAPARALYSES D>S - YELLOWISH LINE, NARROWED RIGHT LEG REFLECTION ZONE

Fig. 168 The patient shown below has peripheral facial paralysis on the right side. The right facial reflection zone is slightly swollen and is of a darker red to brownish color.

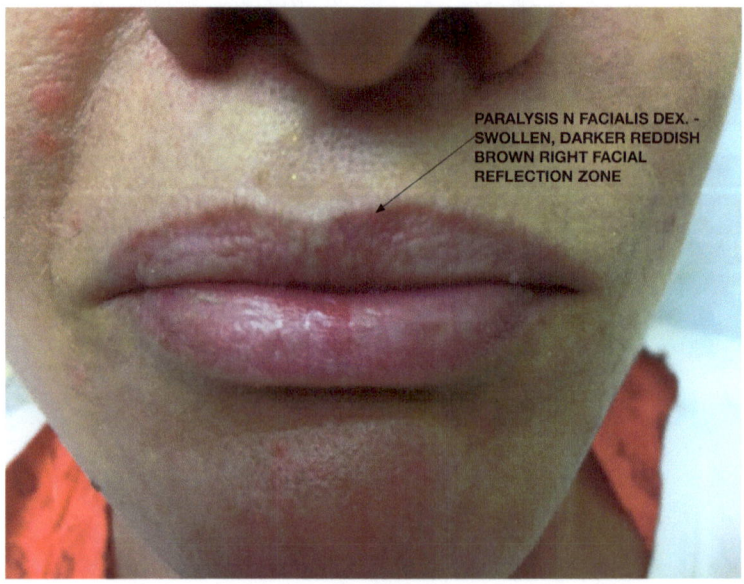

PARALYSIS N FACIALIS DEX. - SWOLLEN, DARKER REDDISH BROWN RIGHT FACIAL REFLECTION ZONE

Fig. 169 The patient below has fibular nerve paralysis of the right leg and disc herniation at L4-L5. The perennial muscles are atrophied, and the patient has no dorsal flexion. The right perennial muscle reflection zone is narrowed with a horizontal fold and is yellowish in color.

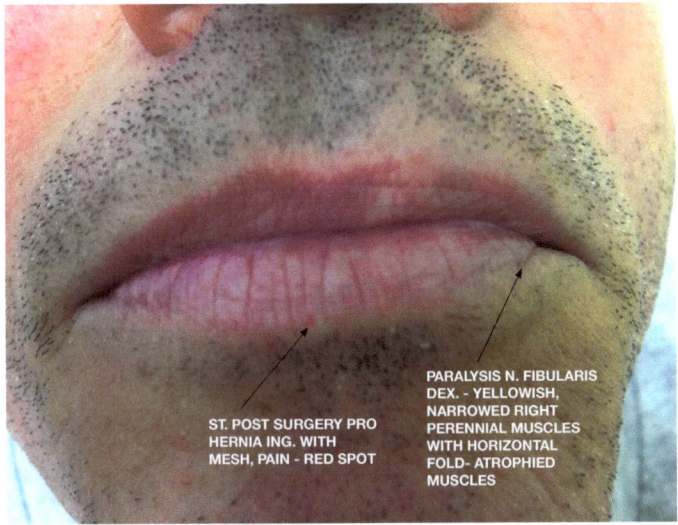

6.5 Tumors of the Nervous System

Fig. 170 The patient below had surgery on the right anterotemporal side for a subdural hematoma. The lip membrane on the right anterotemporal reflection zone has been replaced by skin, is slightly swollen zone, and contains a small pink reddish point.

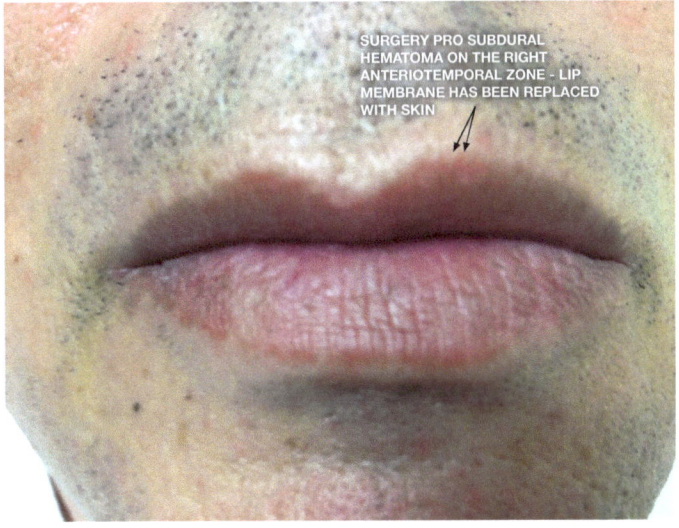

Fig. 171 The patient below had surgery on the right side of the brain to remove a cyst. Afterward, she developed left arm weakness and memory problems. The right reflection zone of the brain contains a yellowish line and brown spots. A similar yellowish line with brown spots can be seen on the left arm reflection zone and indicates a weak left arm.

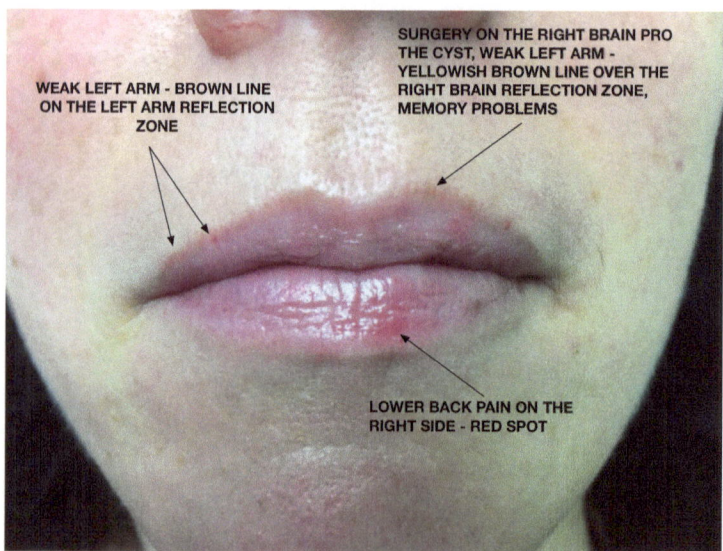

Fig. 172 Two years ago, the patient below had surgery on the right anterotemporal zone for a meningioma. The right anterotemporal reflection zone contains a yellowish bump (arrow).

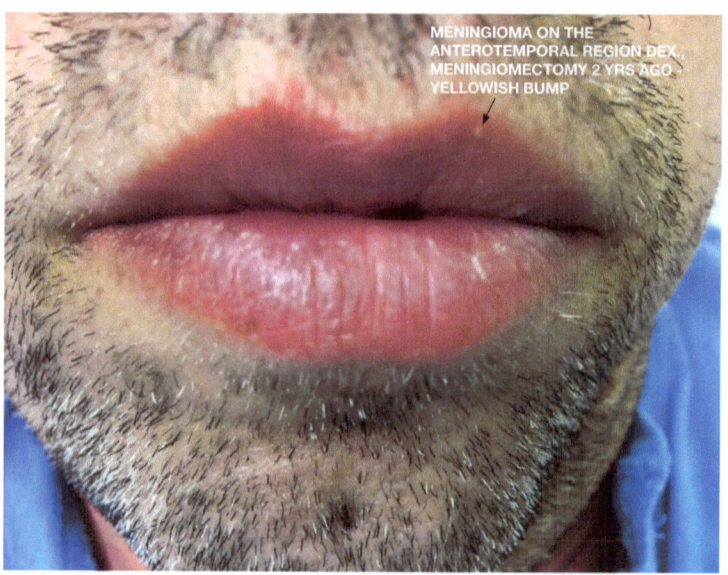

Fig. 173 The patient below has a meningioma on the left fronto-parietal brain zone. The left fronto-parietal brain reflection zone contains a darker point (arrow).

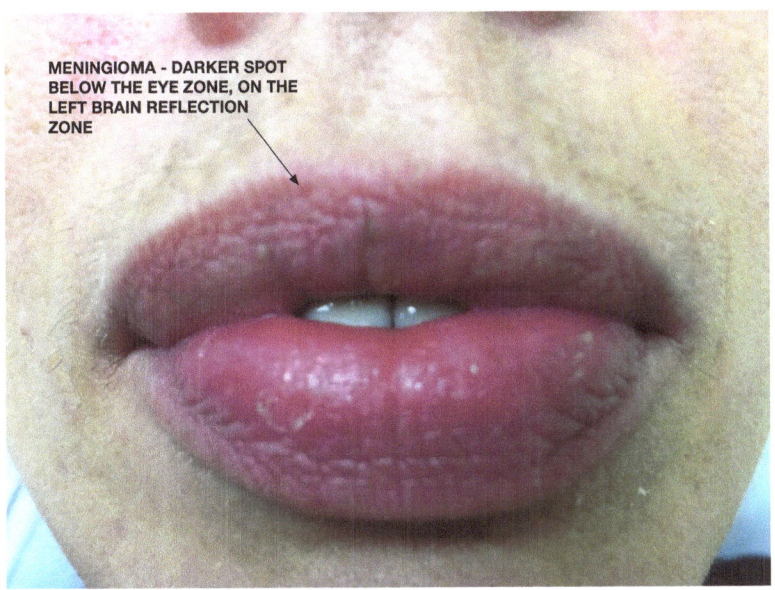

6.6 Eyes

Fig. 174 The patient below had laser surgery for myopia of the right eye and suffered vision loss. The lip membrane of the right eye reflection zone was replaced by skin (arrow).

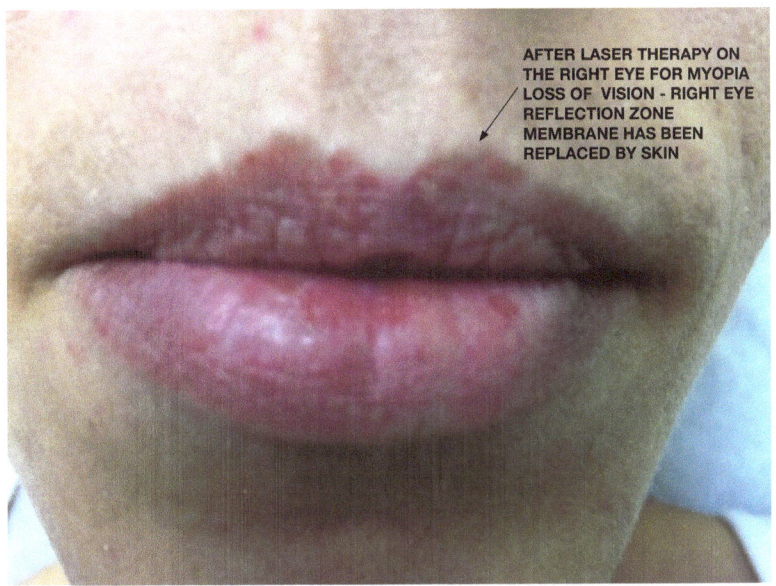

Fig. 175 The patient below has glaucoma that manifested more intensely on right side than the left side. The eye reflection zones are light yellowish in color and contain dark vertical lines.

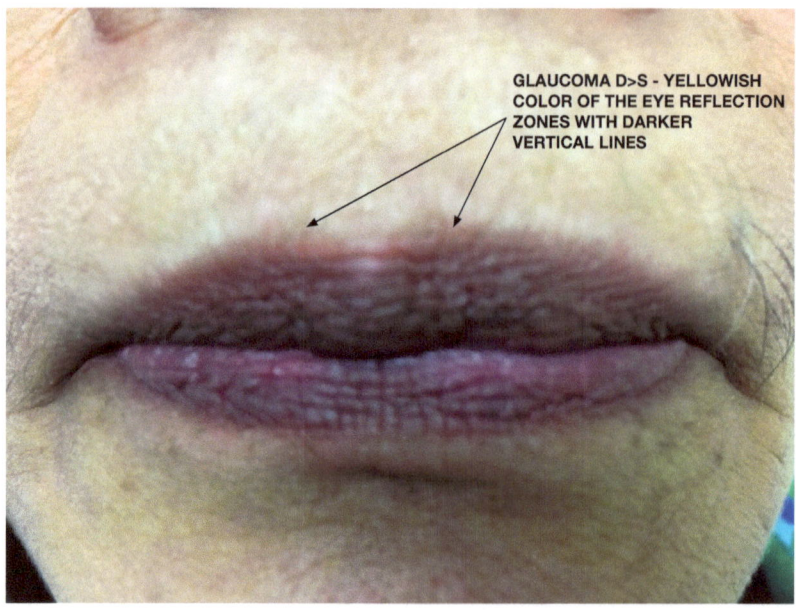

Fig. 176 The patient below has cataracts. The eye reflection zones are a very light yellowish color, and the lip membrane has been replaced by skin.

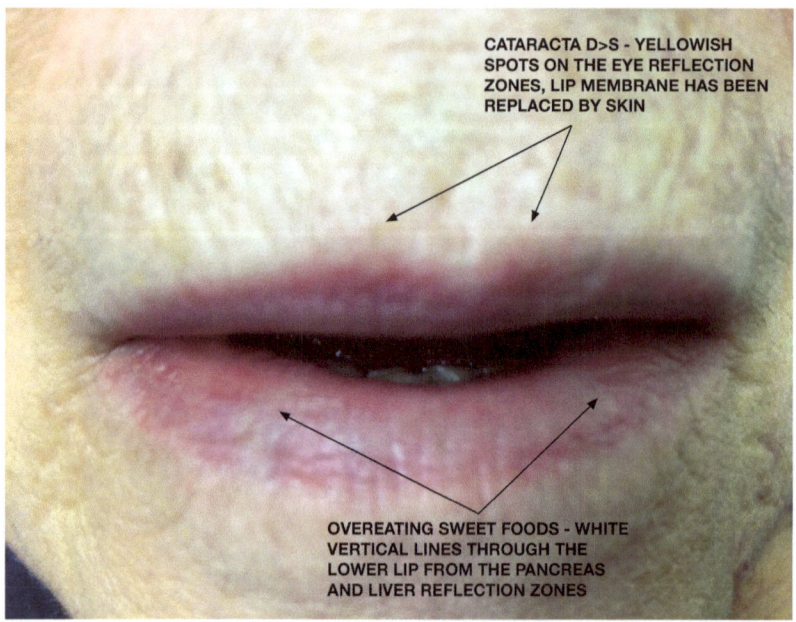

Fig. 177 The patient below had surgery on the lacrimal channels of the eyes. An obstruction of the lacrimal channels caused an increase in eye pressure. Yellowish brown spots can be seen in the eye reflection zones. The right reflection zone is larger than the left.

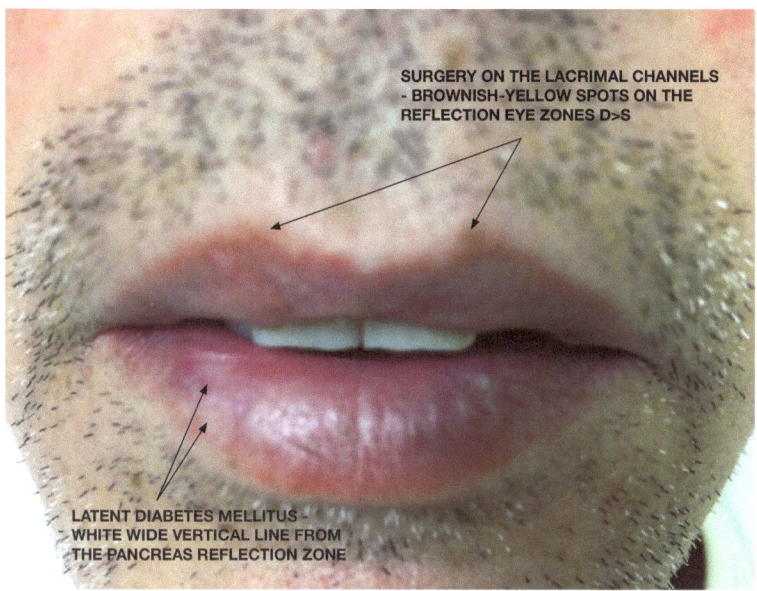

Fig. 178 During childhood, the patient below experienced trauma to the right eye from sun exposure that resulted in myopia. The right eye reflection zone contains a large brown spot that has spread above the reflection zone. Part of the lip membrane in the right eye reflection zone has been replaced by skin.

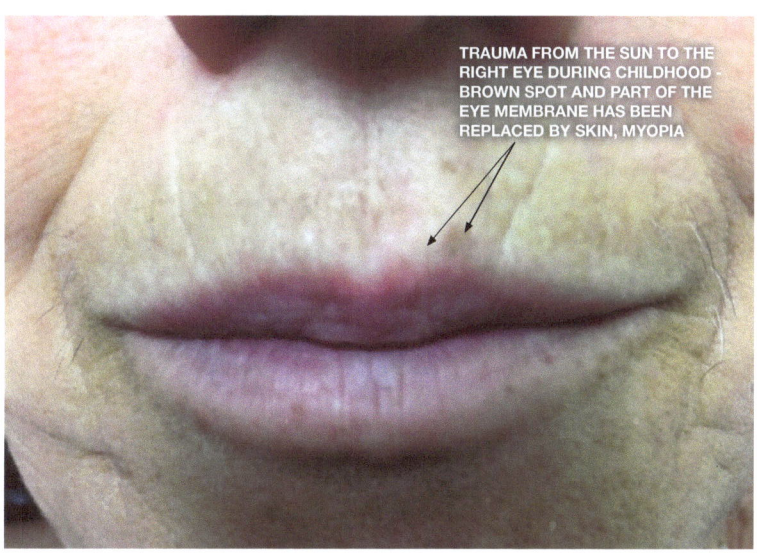

Fig. 179 The patient below has lens deformation in the right eye. The right eye reflection zone contains a red spot.

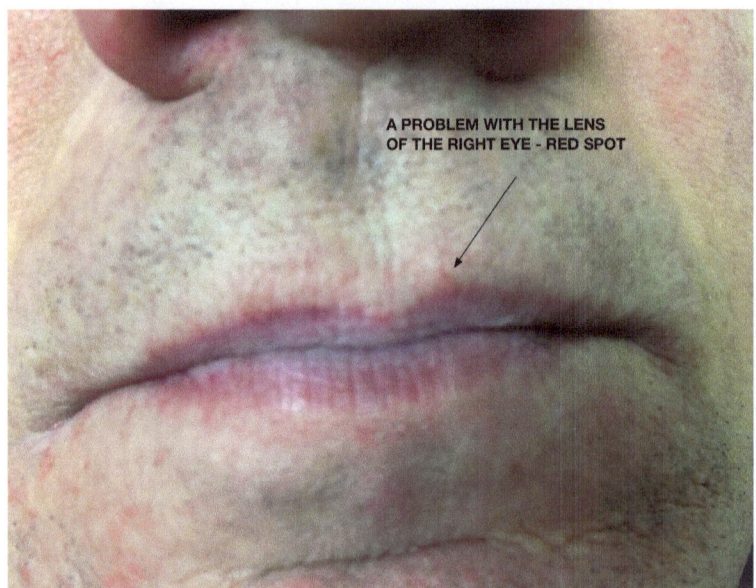

Fig. 180 The patient below experienced loss of vision in the left eye and myopia of the right eye after a traumatic incident. The lip membrane of the right eye reflection zone has been replaced by skin. Vertical yellowish lines starting at the eye reflection zones travel to above the upper lip.

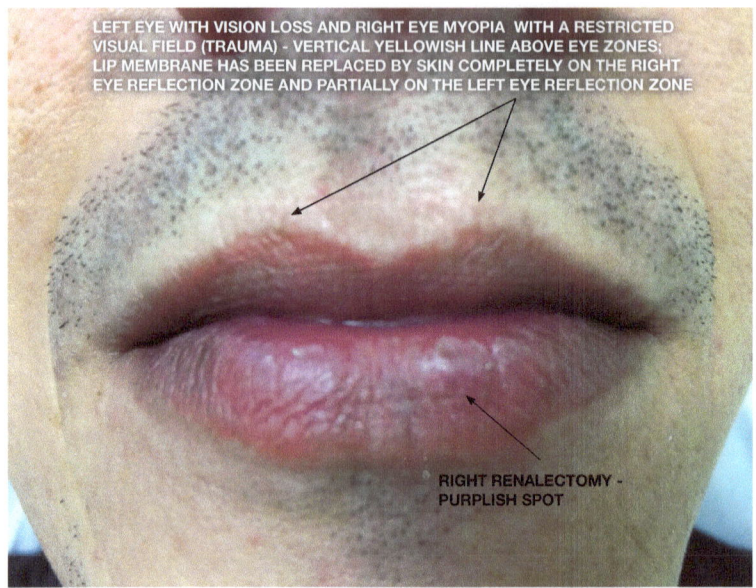

Fig. 181 The patient below experienced a severe trauma to the right eye with consequent myopia, fifteen years ago. The lip membrane of the right eye reflection zone has been replaced by skin. There is a vertical white line stretching from the right eye reflection zone to above the upper lip.

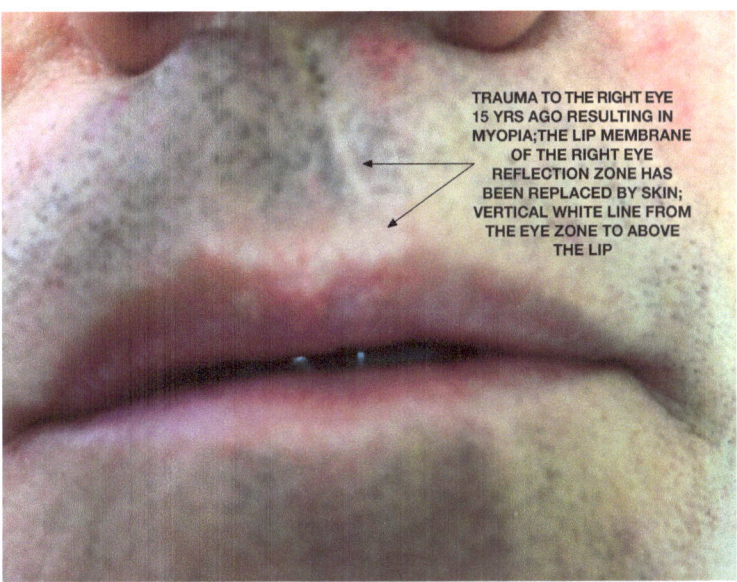

Fig. 182 The patient below experienced trauma to the left eye twenty years ago. The red spot has moved directly above the left eye reflection zone to the skin over the years.

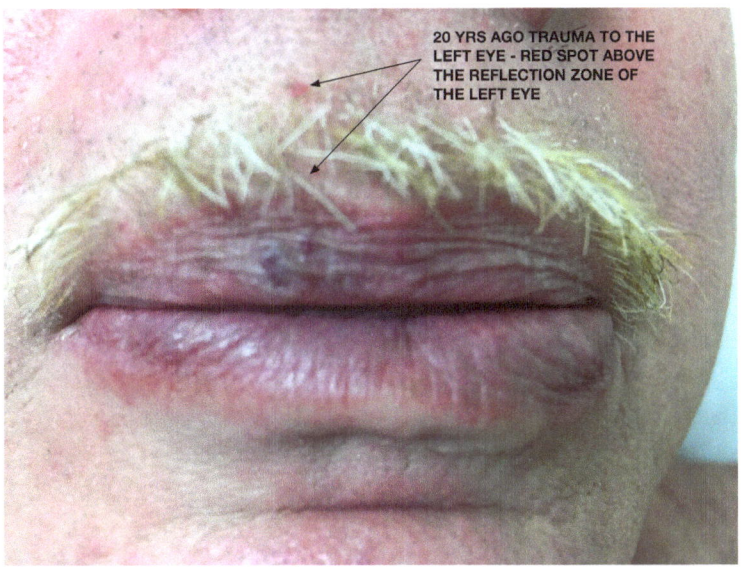

Fig. 183 The patient below had laser surgery on the left eye six years ago. The red spot has moved directly above the left eye reflection zone over the years.

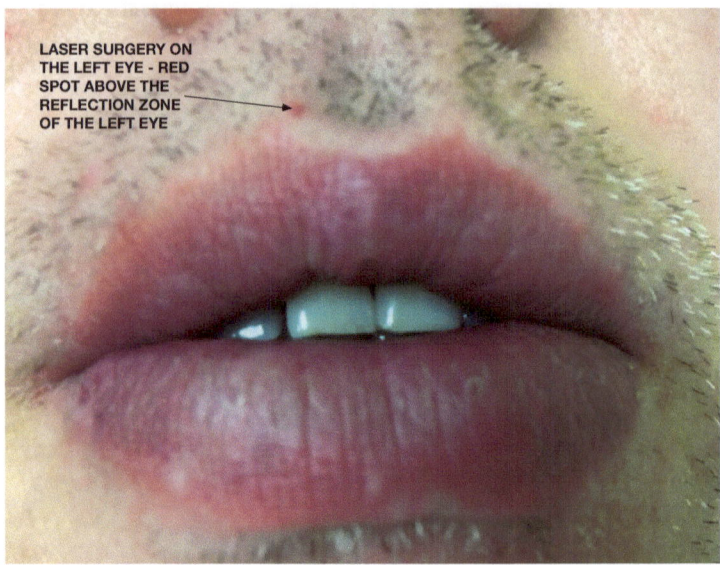

Fig. 184 The patient below has chronic uveitis that manifests more in the left eye than the right eye, and is caused by chronic sinusitis. The process of replacement of the lip membrane with skin in the eye, throat, and sinuses reflection zones is ongoing. The left sinus reflection zone contains a red spot indicating an active infectious process (middle arrow).

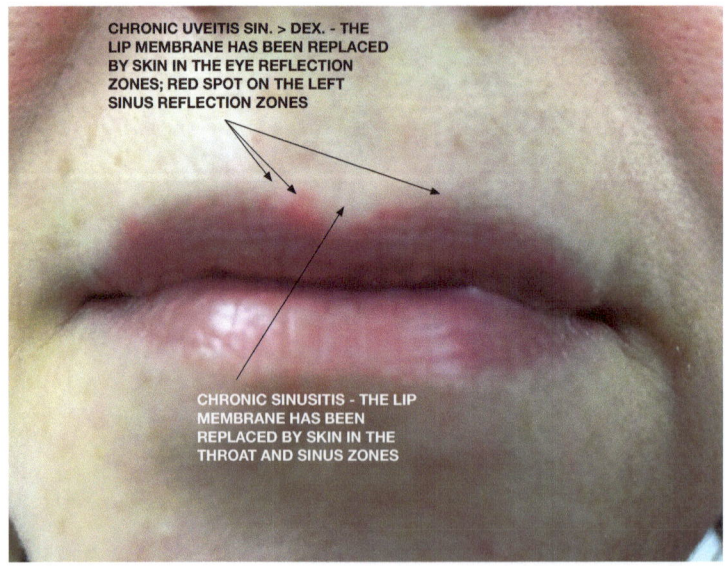

Fig. 185 Eleven years ago the patient below had a retinal ablation of the right eye. There is a brown spot above the left eye reflection zone and partial replacement of the lip membrane with skin in the right eye reflection zone.

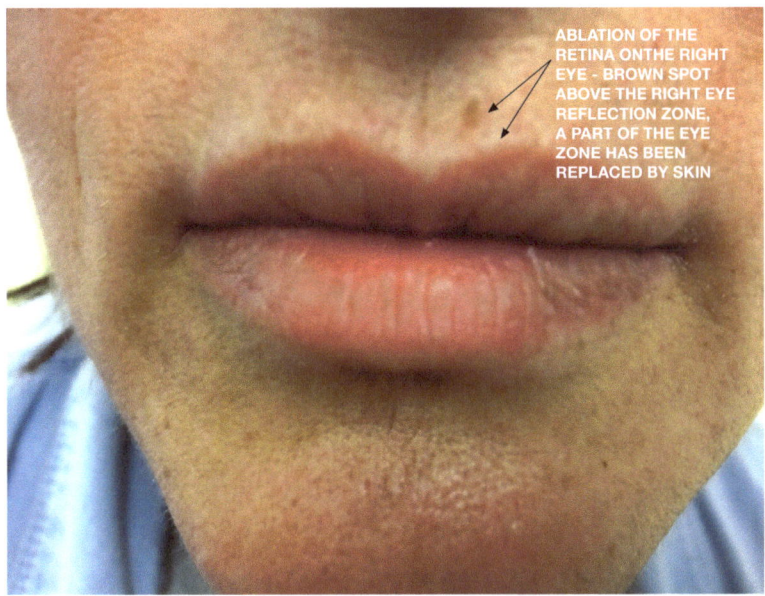

Fig. 186 Twenty years ago the patient below had an ablation of the retina on the right eye. There are two brown spots above the right eye reflection zone and the lip membrane has been slightly replaced by skin.

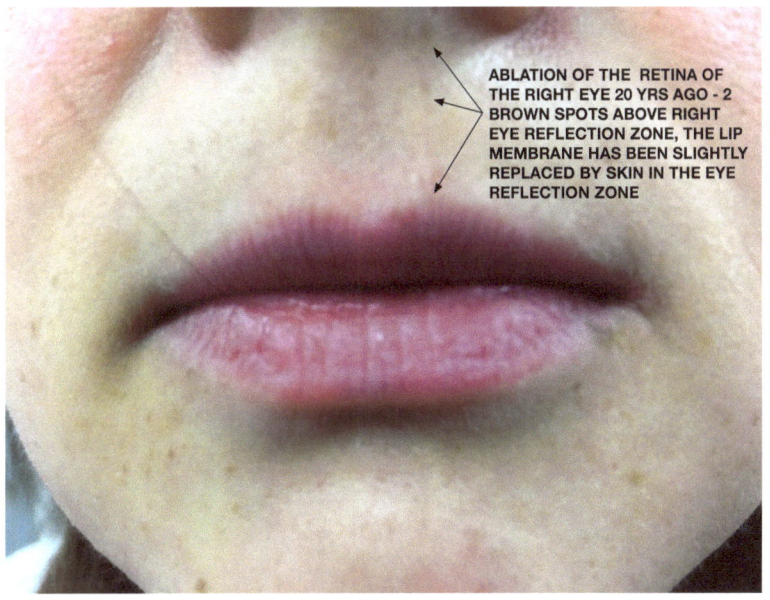

7. Pathologic Processes of the Musculoskeletal System

7.1 Fractures. Traumas

Fig. 188 The patient in the photograph below fractured the second cervical vertebra in a car accident. A red spot formed on the neck reflection zone (arrow).

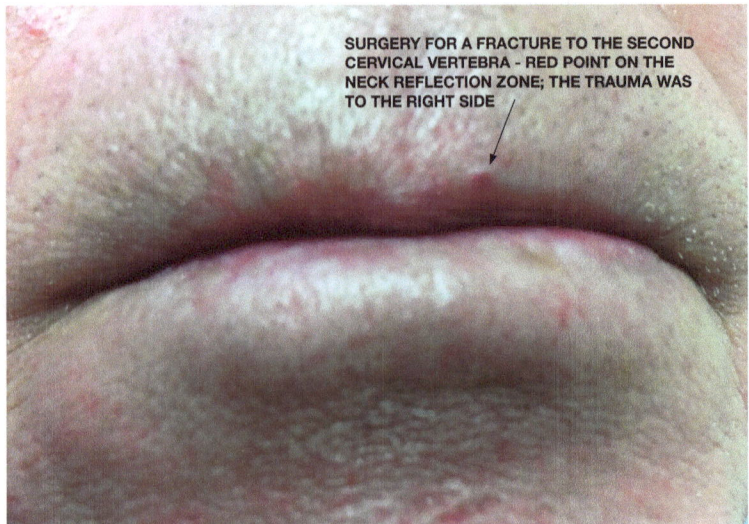

Fig. 189 The patient below experienced trauma to the right knee that involved tearing of the medial meniscus and a fracture to the patella six years ago. The right knee reflection zone contains brown spots that are connected to the red point below the lip. The red point migrated out of the knee reflection zone over time.

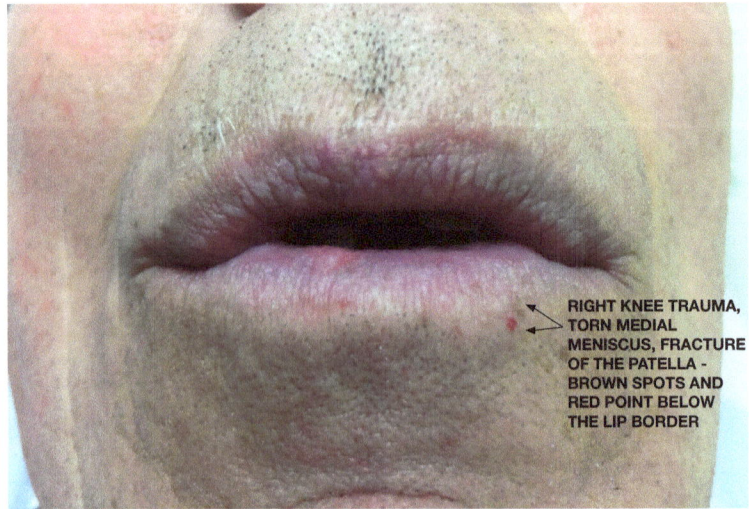

Fig. 190 The patient in the photograph below experienced a severe trauma to the right knee twenty-seven years ago. The right knee reflection zone contains a dark spot and there is a yellowish bump below the lower lip (arrows).

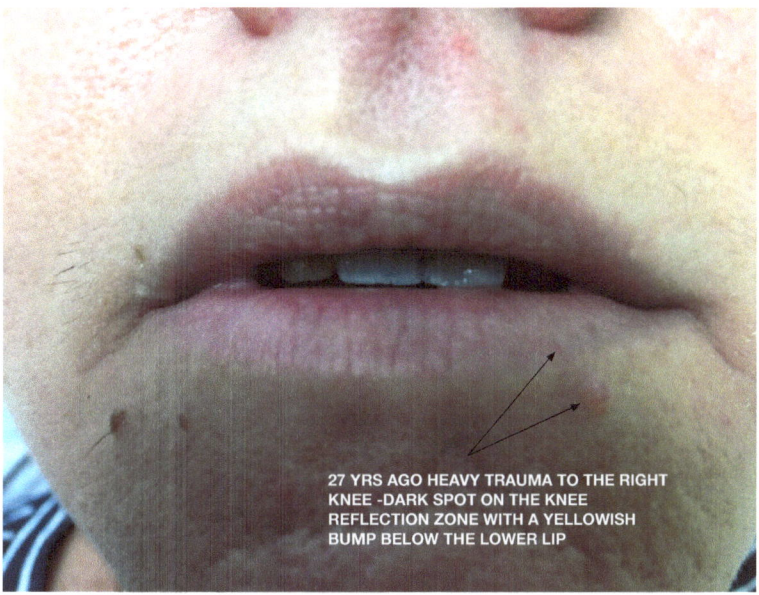

Fig. 191 Twenty years ago, a bullet lodged in the lower part of the right hip of the patient below that could not be removed surgically. The right hip reflection zone contains a purplish bump (arrow).

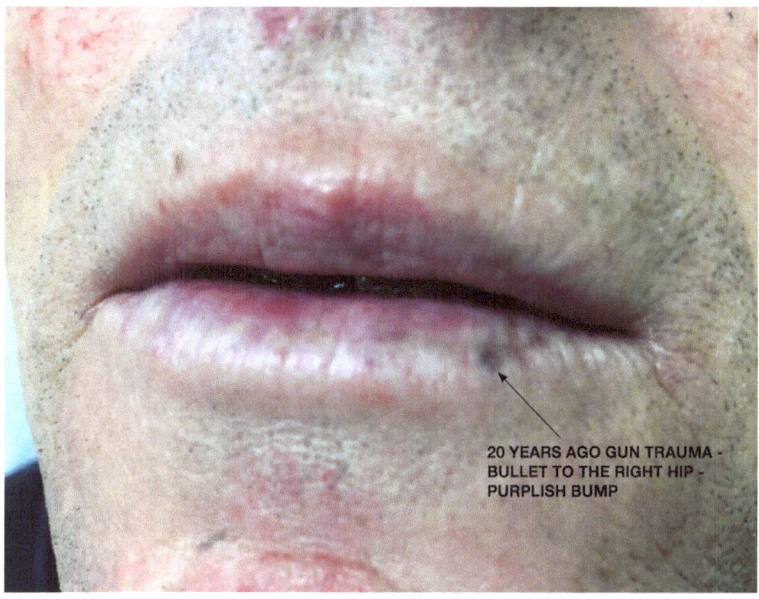

Lip Diagnostics

Fig. 192 The patient below suffered multiple fractures to the right femur, tibia, fibula, and ankle after a car accident. The right leg reflection zone contains multiple white vertical lines indicating the position of the fractures (arrows).

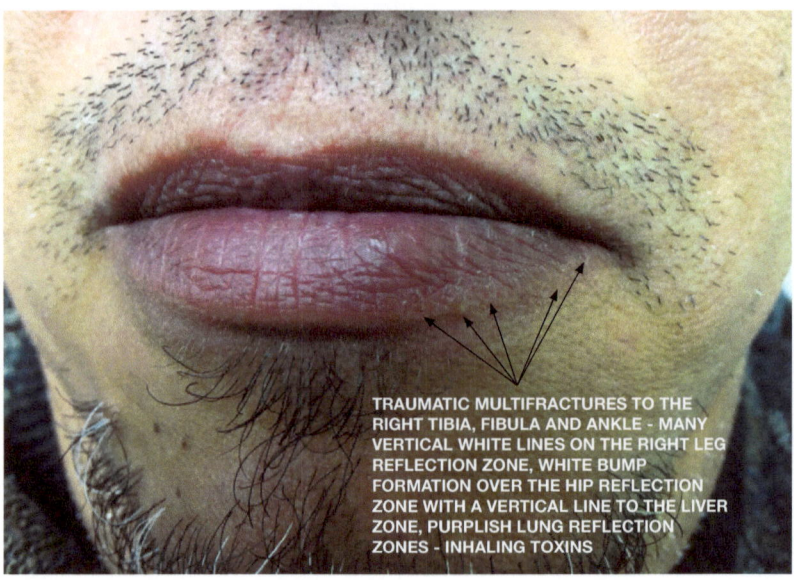

TRAUMATIC MULTIFRACTURES TO THE RIGHT TIBIA, FIBULA AND ANKLE - MANY VERTICAL WHITE LINES ON THE RIGHT LEG REFLECTION ZONE, WHITE BUMP FORMATION OVER THE HIP REFLECTION ZONE WITH A VERTICAL LINE TO THE LIVER ZONE, PURPLISH LUNG REFLECTION ZONES - INHALING TOXINS

Fig. 193 The patient pictured below experienced a fracture to the right fibula five years ago. The right fibula reflection zone contains a white vertical line (arrow).

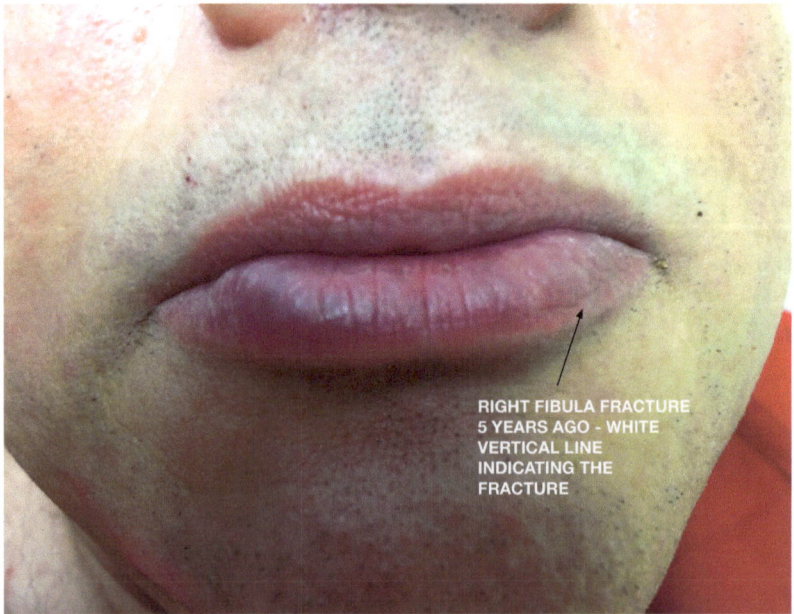

RIGHT FIBULA FRACTURE 5 YEARS AGO - WHITE VERTICAL LINE INDICATING THE FRACTURE

Fig. 194.1.2 The patient below experienced serious trauma with fractures to five ribs on the left and right side. Additionally, the cartilage of his left knee was surgically removed thirteen years ago. The chest reflection zones contain transversal lines and the left knee reflection zone contains a purplish spot (arrows).

Fig. 194.1

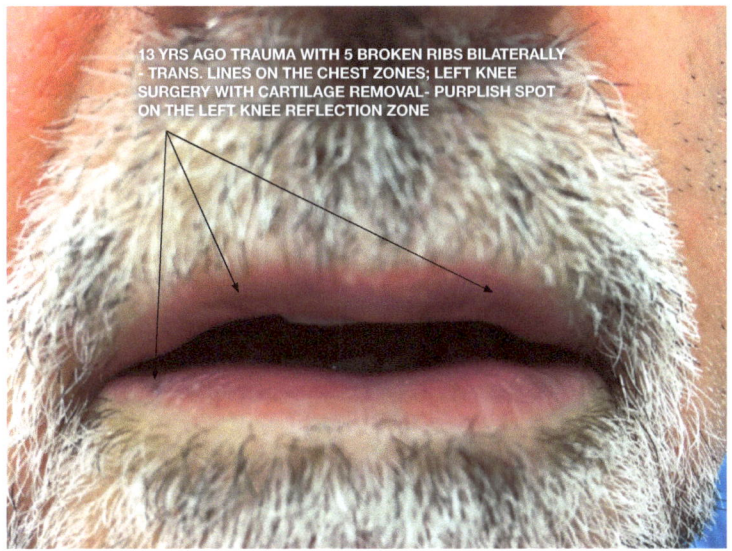

Fig. 194.2

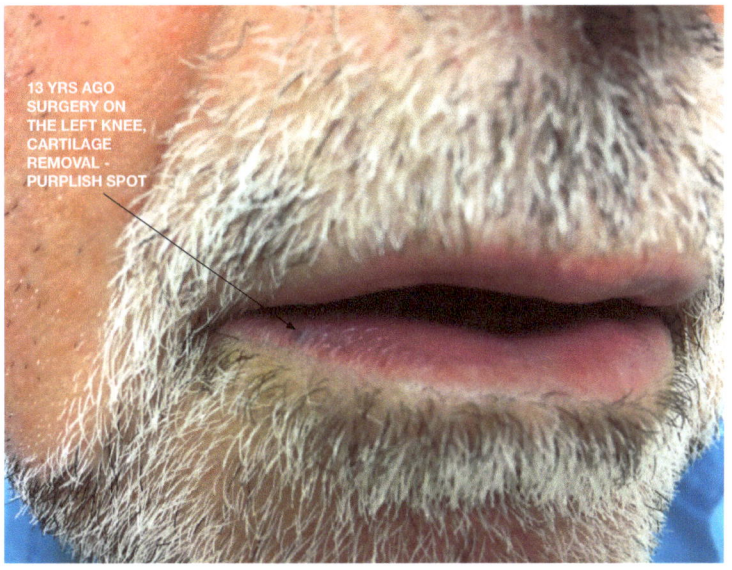

Lip Diagnostics

Fig. 195 The patient below sustained a trauma to the left leg that caused a partial tearing of the medial meniscus and overstretching of the medial collateral ligament of the knee joint. Additionally, he is experiencing muscle ache and pain in the hip joint. The left leg reflection zone contains red spots in the areas corresponding to the hip joint, hip muscles, and knee joint.

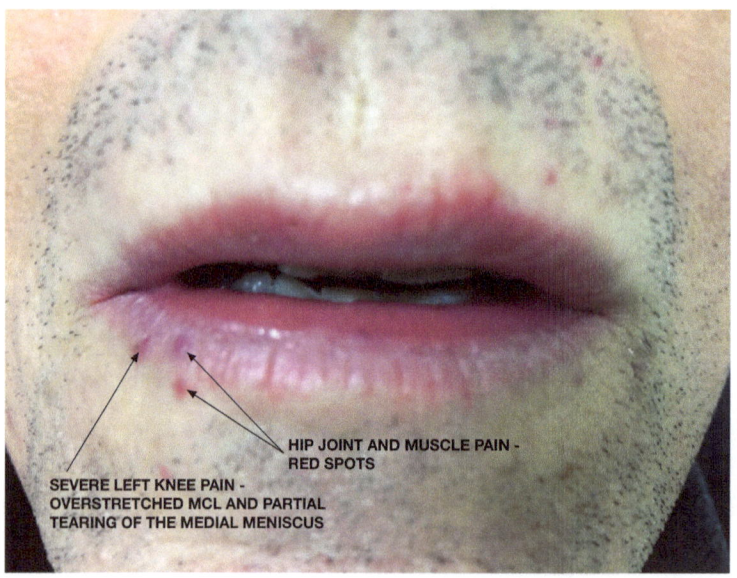

Fig. 196 The patient below experienced severe trauma to the right hip joint eight years ago. The right hip joint reflection zone contains a red spot. There is a brown spot below the lip border.

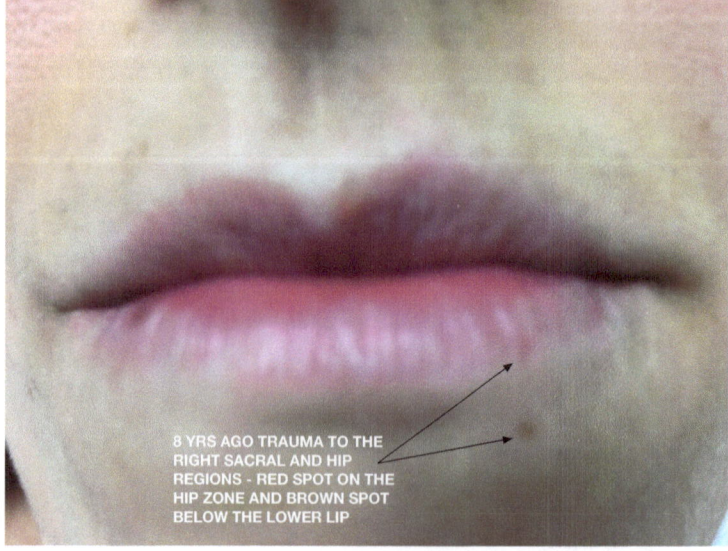

New Reflection Zones of the Human Organs on the Lips

Fig. 197 Currently, the patient pictured below is experiencing left knee pain. Twenty-three years ago, the patient suffered a trauma to the lower back that resulted in disc protrusions and dislocation of the lumbar region of the spine. Twenty-seven years ago, a bone fragment lodged in the joint when he fractured his right wrist and left elbow. The left knee reflection zone contains a white spot, which is indicative of pain. The left lumbar reflection zone contains a red point indicating the disc protrusion. The right wrist reflection zone contains a vertical red line, and the lip membrane has been replaced with skin. The left elbow reflection zone contains a white bump with a small red vertical line showing the bone fragment lodged in the joint.

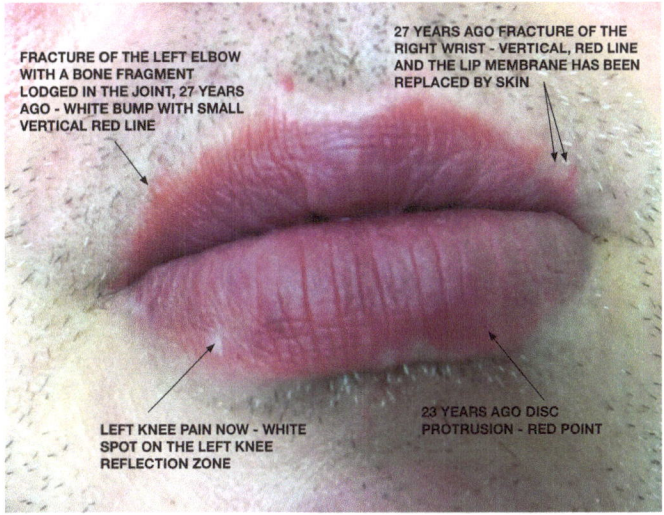

Fig. 198 The patient below has had a dental procedure. A tooth on the left lower side of the mouth was extracted and replaced by an implant. The reflection zone corresponding to the teeth on the left side of the mouth contains a red triangular spot.

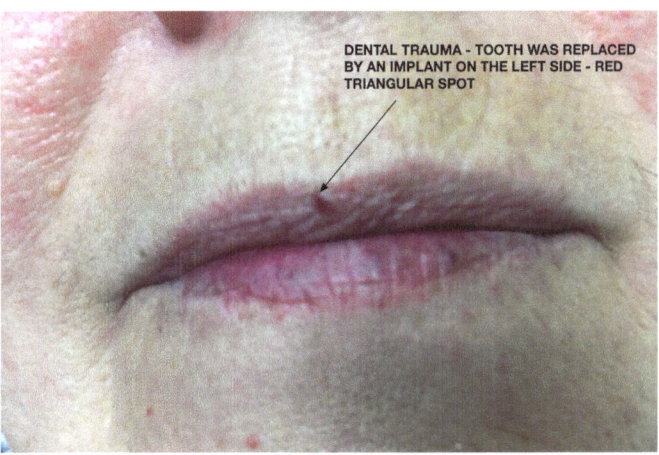

Lip Diagnostics

Fig. 199 The patient below experienced trauma to the left frontal and anterior-temporal region of the head many years ago. The left frontal and anterior-temporal reflection regions contain a large white spot (arrows).

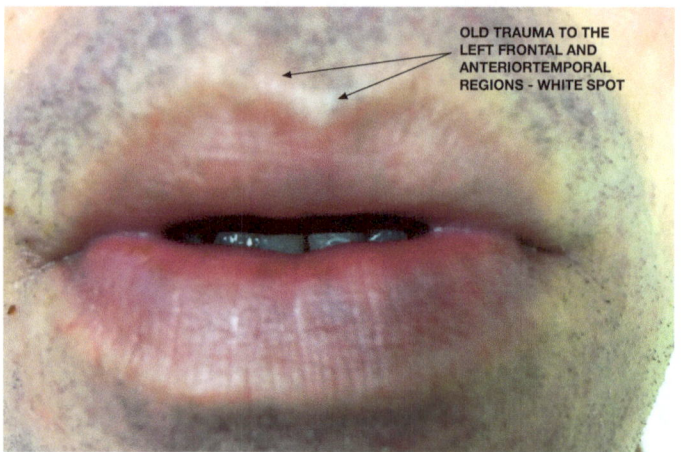

7.2 Arthrosoarthritis

Fig. 200 The patient below has a thirty year history of rheumatoid arthritis. She had a bad case of tonsillitis due to Streptococcus aureus and had surgery to remove her tonsils. Currently she has immobilization of the right humeral and elbow joints; a dislocated right hip joint; insufficiency of the mitral, aortal and tricuspid valves; glomerulonephritis; and hypertonia. The right humeral reflection zone contains a brown spot. There is a reddish –yellow bump on the right elbow reflection zone, and the right hip reflection zone contains a red bump.

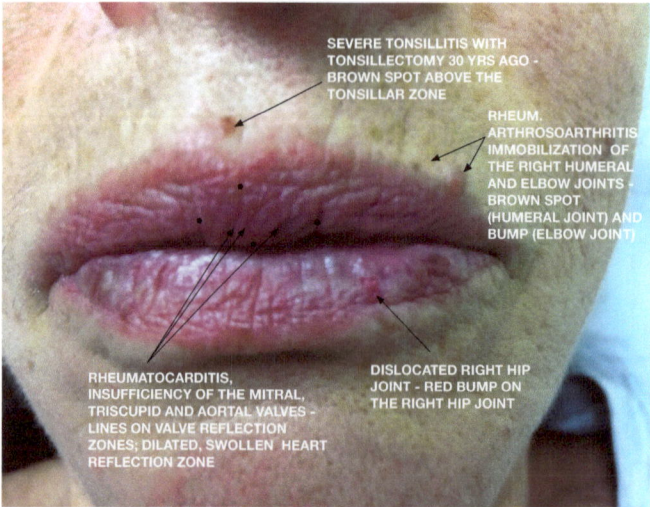

130   *Manifestations of the Diseases on the Lip Organ Zones*

Fig. 201 The patient below has a long history of rheumatism and is experiencing severe pain in the lumbosacral region and the right hip joint that radiates throughout the leg. Additionally, she suffers from a swollen and painful knee, and swollen ankle joints. The reflection zones corresponding to the lumbosacral region and right leg joint contain purplish brown spots and brown lines (arrows).

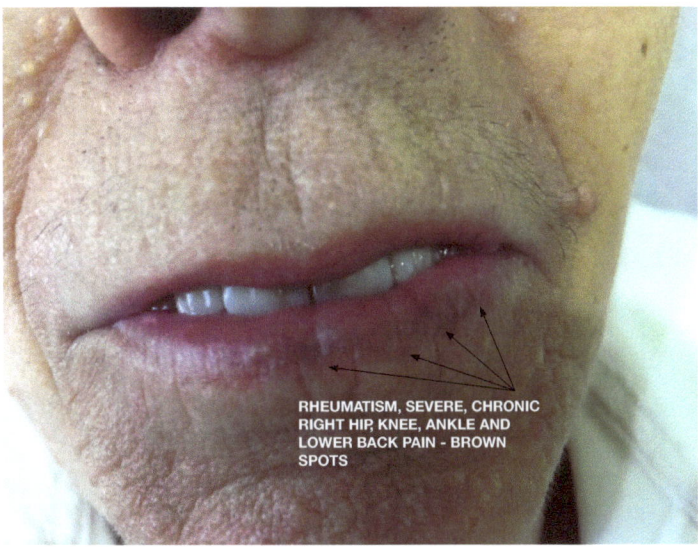

Fig. 202 The patient below has chronic pain in the neck, arm, and leg joints due to osteoarthritis. The neck reflection zone contains brown spots, and the arm and leg reflection zones show vertical folds above the lip borders.

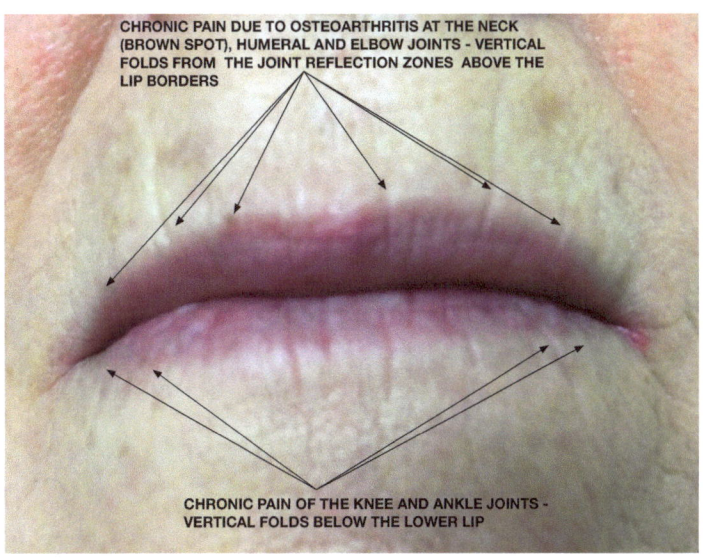

Fig. 203 The patient below has severe chronic pain of the right humeral joint due to osteoarthritis. The right humeral joint reflection zone contains a brown spot and there is a large red spot above the lip border.

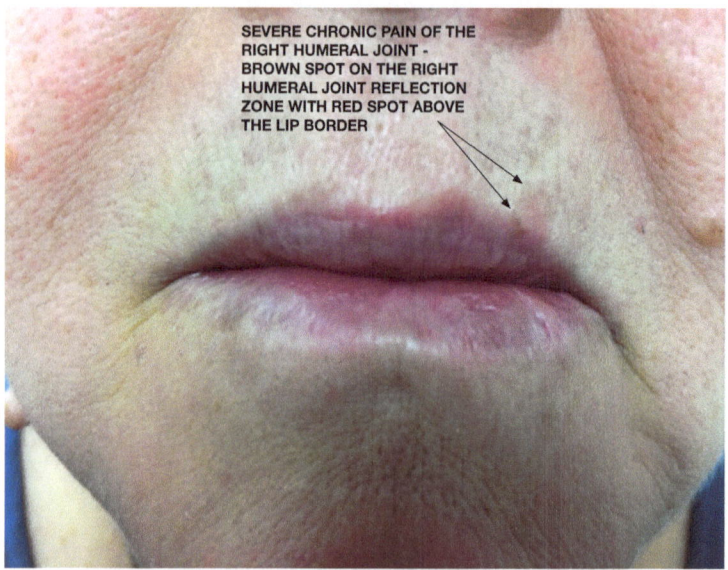

Fig. 204 The patient below has a long history of arthroso-arthritis of the right hip and knee and has had hip replacement surgery. The right hip joint reflection zone contains a transversal line, and the right knee reflection zone contains a purplish bump (arrows).

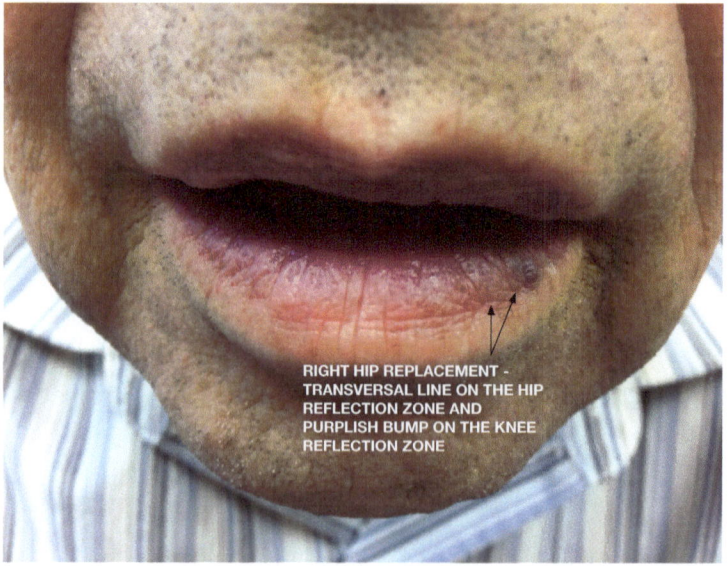

Fig. 205 Ten years ago the patient pictured below experienced severe pain, swelling, and nodule formation on the left elbow joint following an infectious process. There is a brown spot above the left elbow reflection zone (arrow). The left elbow reflection zone is light yellowish in color and contains a vertical fold to the brown spot above the upper lip.

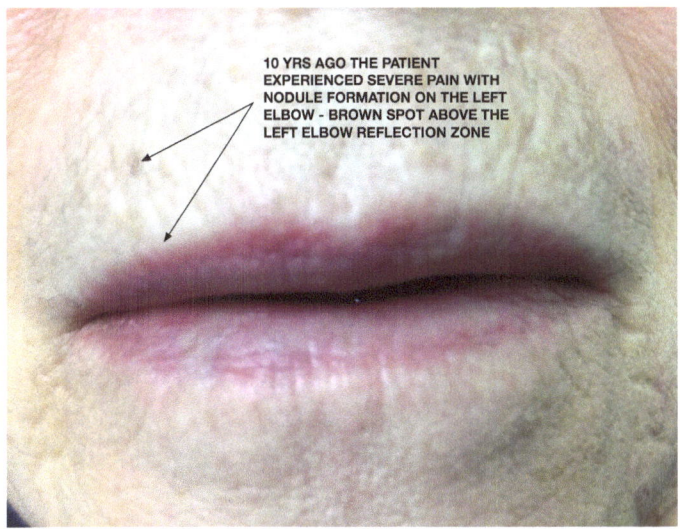

7.3 Osteochondrosis

Fig. 206 The patient below has severe pain that starts in the lower back and spreads through the right leg to the toes. She has a disc protrusion at L4-5 and L5-S1 that causes radiculopathy at the fifth lumbar and first sacral nerves. A thick white line runs through the right leg reflection zone (arrows).

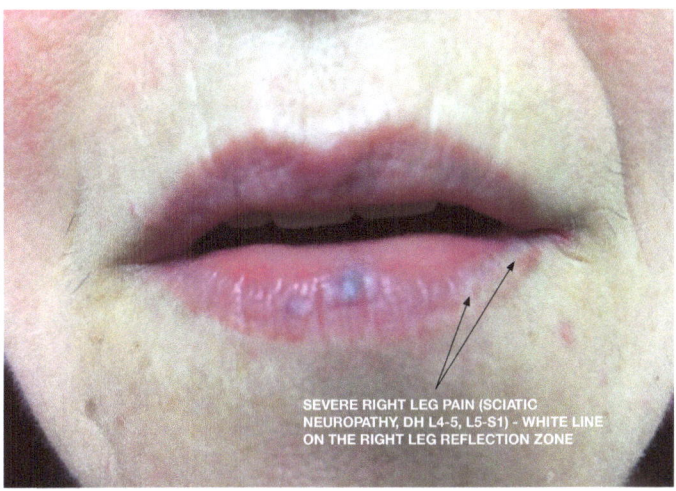

Fig. 207 The patient below has a chlamydia infection of the prostate that spread to the sciatic nerve and causes strong burning pain in the lower back and the right gluteal region. The prostate reflection zone contains a yellowish spot and a yellowish line connecting the prostate and lower back regions. The right sacral and gluteal reflection zones contain a similar yellowish spot as well as red spots.

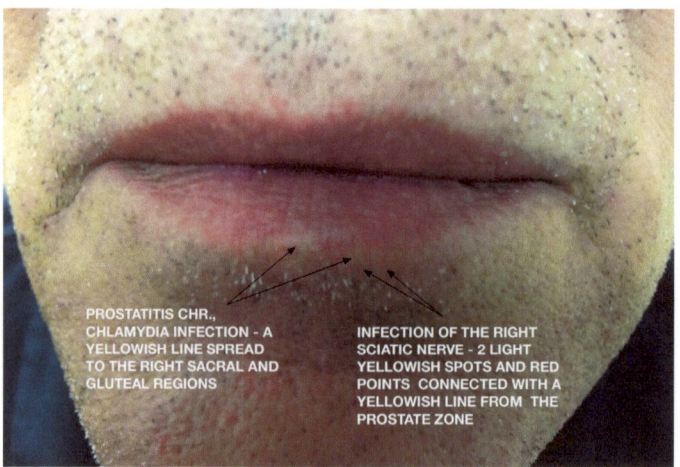

Fig. 208 The patient below has scoliosis of the right lumbar region, and disc protrusion at L3-L4, L4-L5 and L5-S1. The patient is experiencing severe lumbar pain that restricts his movements. The pain has spread through the right leg. The right lumbar reflection zone contains a curved yellowish line indicating scoliosis (left arrow). There are miniscule red spots at DH L4-5, L5-S1 (middle arrow). The right leg reflection zone contains a yellowish line (right arrow). After 30 seconds of laser therapy applied over the tiny red spots, the patient experienced a significant reduction to the pain and was able to walk unaided and lie down on the examination bed.

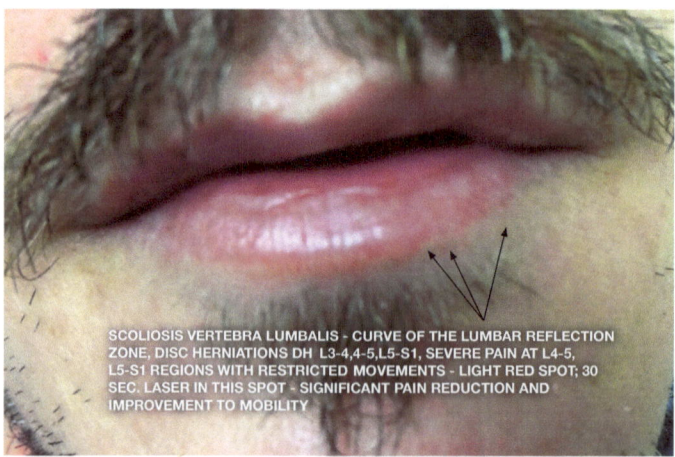

Fig. 209 The patient below has osteochondrosis in the cervical and lumbar regions of the vertebra that causes severe neck pain and numbness in the arms. The right side of the neck is more painful than the left. The same is true of the lower back. The neck reflection zones contain red spots on the areas corresponding to the most affected discs. The arm reflection zones are slightly swollen and are yellowish in color. The right lumbar reflection zone contains a large red spot, which migrated below the lower lip border. There are brown spots far above the neck reflection zones, which are a sign of a long term degenerative process.

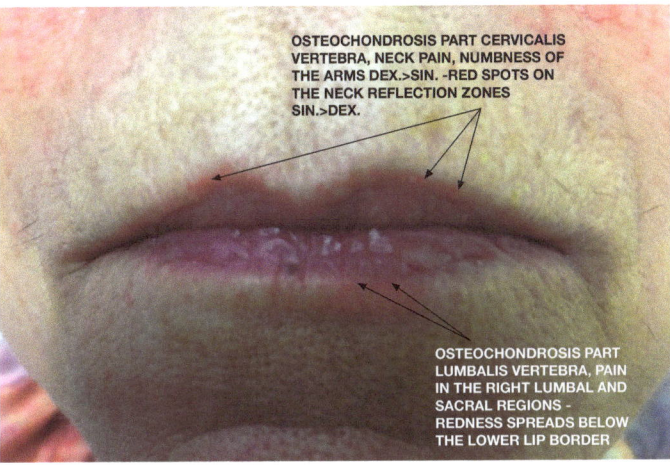

8. Pathologic Processes of the Skin

Fig. 210 The patient below has veal-skin (vitiligo) that started on the fingers and toes. The foot and hand reflection zones contain large white spots where the skin has been discolored (arrows).

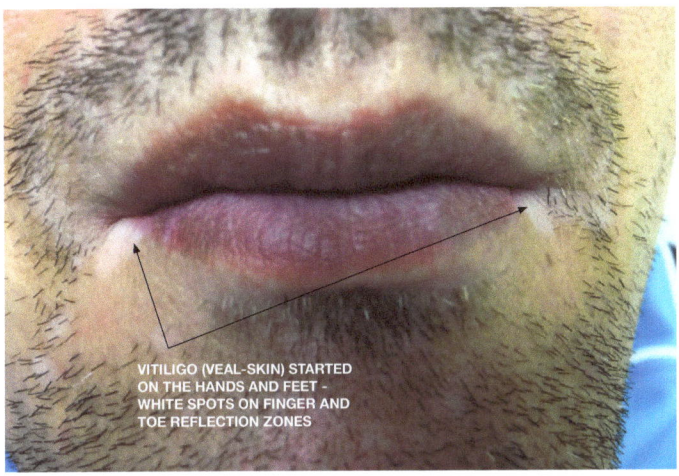

Fig. 211 The patient has psoriatic plaques on the right hand and foot. The right hand and foot reflection zones contain white spots and the epidermis is peeling (hyperkeratosis).

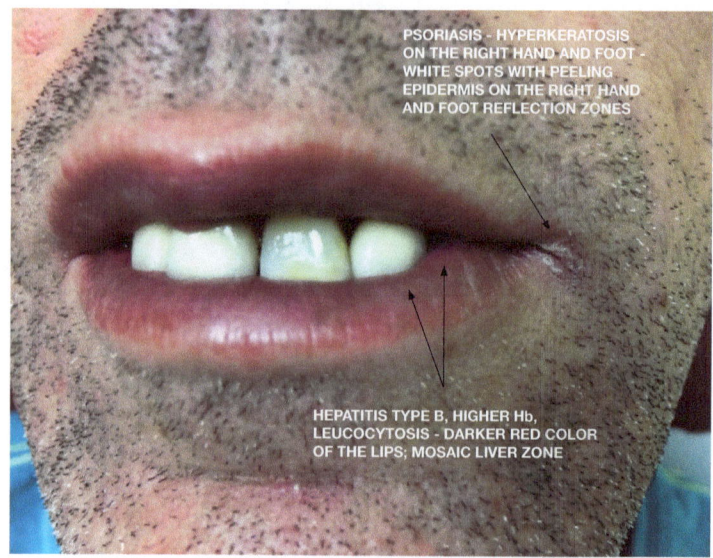

Fig. 212 The patient below developed a strong allergic reaction to cleaning detergents on the hands and forearms. The skin is swollen, cracked, and very itchy. The hand and forearm reflection zones contain dark lines and spots. The corresponding zones are slightly swollen, and the spleen reflection zone is swollen, as well. Vertical lines run from the spleen reflection zones through the lower lip.

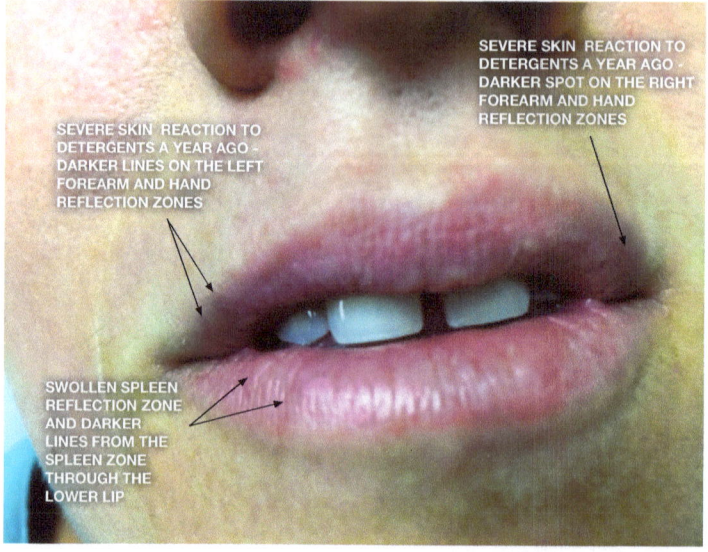

Fig. 213 The patient pictured below has multiple lipomatous nodes beneath the skin of the arms and legs. The skin reflection zones of the arms and legs contain many small yellowish bumps on the lower lip borders (arrows).

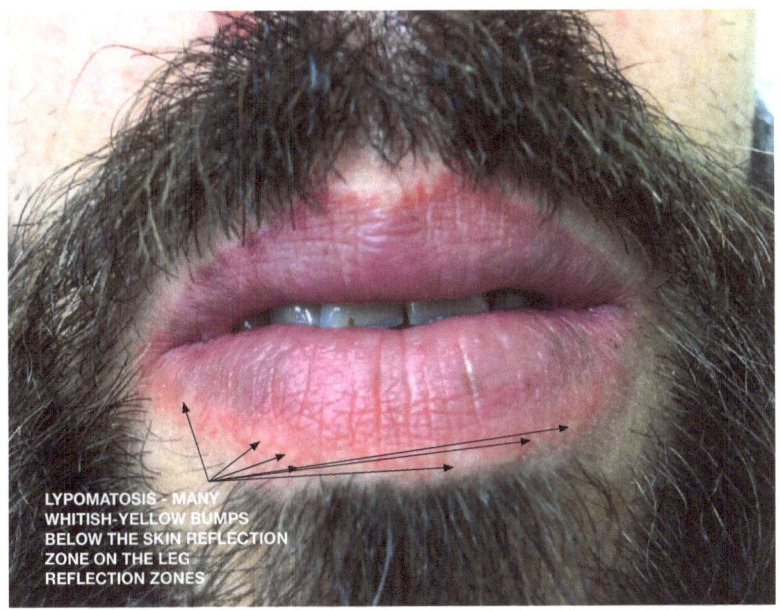

SECTION VII

LIP THERAPY

Lips are useful not only for diagnostic purposes but also for therapy. The application of a soft laser on the reflection zones of the organs has a very fast and strong painkilling effect. In my practice, I have seen many patients with pain in various organs or parts of the body who experienced a reduction or full cessation of pain symptoms after 20-30 seconds of laser therapy.

Laser acupuncture has a long history, going back more than fifty years. It has proved useful in treating hypertonia, inflammatory bowel diseases, trauma, and arthrosoarthitis of the joints, as well as metabolic diseases. There have been reports of successfully stopping epileptic convulsions by focusing a laser beam on the upper lip of the patient at the onset of a seizure. [24, 25, 26]

SECTION VIII

LITERATURE

1. shutterstock_773922037.jpg
2. shutterstock_763933174.jpg; shutterstock_647309011-2.jpg
3. https://en.wikipedia.org/wiki/Iridology
4. Reflection zones on the tongue (editor map)
5. shutterstock_294226676.jpg
6. Guyton, Arthur, C., Hall, John, E., 2006,Textbook of Medical Physiology, eleventh edition, ELSEVIER SAUNDERS, ISBN-13: 978-0-7216-0240-0
7. homonculous.jpg; rendered.jpg
8. https://tcmwiki.com/wiki/governor-vessel; https://tcmwiki.com/wiki/conception-vessel
9. Law Smith, Miriam J.; Deady, Denis K.; Moore, Fhionna R.; Jones, Benedict C.; Cornwell, R. Elisabeth; Stirrat, Michael; Lawson, Jamie F.; Feinberg, David R.; Perrett, David I. (2011-09-21). "Maternal tendencies in women are associated with estrogen levels and facial femininity". *Hormones and Behavior.* **61** *(1): 12–6. doi:10.1016/j.yhbeh.2011.09.005. PMID 21983237*
10. https://en.wikipedia.org/wiki/Lip
11. Miller-Keane Encyclopedia and Dictionary of Medicine, Nursing, and Allied Health, Seventh Edition. © 2003 by Saunders, an imprint of Elsevier, Inc. All rights reserved
12. Dorland's Medical Dictionary for Health Consumers. © 2007 by Saunders, an imprint of Elsevier, Inc. All rights reserved
13. Mosby's Dental Dictionary, 2nd edition. © 2008 Elsevier, Inc. All rights reserved

14. WebMD, http:// www.webmd.com/ a-to-z-guides/ folic-acid-deficiency-anemia-symptoms
15. Mayo Clinic, http:// www.mayoclinic.com/health/vitamin-b2/ns patient-riboflavin
16. https://www.webmd.com/a-to-z-guides/oral-herpes
17. https://www.mouthhealthy.org/en/az-topics/s/sexually-transmitted-disease
18. https://www.mycarmex.com/wp-content/uploads/LipBook.pdf
19. https://www.healthline.com/health/mucous-cyst
20. https://www.colgate.com › ... › Conditions › Mouth Sores & Infections
21. Molnar L, Ronay P, Tapolcsanyi L. Carcinoma of the lip. Analysis of the material of 25 years. *Oncology* 1974; 29:101-21
22. Bridges, Lillian, 2012, Face Reading in Chinese Medicine, second edition, CHURCHILL LIVINGSTONE ELSEVIER, ISBN 9780702043147
23. Щекин, Георгий, Б., 2004, Визуална Психодиагностика, Фабер, ISBN 954-775-400-9
24. H. Gris and W. Dick, The New Soviet Psychic Diiscoveries (New York: Warner Books, 1978), p. 397
25. Hecker,H-U. And Steveling, A., Microsystems Acupuncture: The omlete Guide: Ear – Scalp – Mouth – Hand, Thieme, 2011
26. Henry. R., Laser-Quantum Acupuncture and Therapy, Salem Author Services, 2017

GLOSSARY OF MEDICAL TERMS

Arrhythmia: A condition in which the heart beats with an irregular or abnormal rhythm.

Arthrosoarthritis: Arthritis is an umbrella term used to describe several conditions that cause inflammation in the joints. In some cases, the inflammation can also affect your skin, muscles, and organs. Arthrosis is another name for osteoarthritis the most common type of arthritis.

Biliary Cirrhosis: Primary biliary cirrhosis is an autoimmune disease of the liver. It results from a slow, progressive destruction of the small bile ducts of the liver, causing bile and other toxins to build up in the liver.

Bilirubin: An orange-yellow pigment that occurs normally when part of the red blood cells break down. The liver removes bilirubin from the blood and changes its chemical make-up so that most of it is excreted as bile.

BUN: Blood urea nitrogen: A measure of the urea level in blood. Diseases that compromise the function of the kidney frequently lead to increased BUN levels.

Cataracts: A cataract is a clouding of the eye's natural lens, which lies behind the iris and the pupil. Cataracts are the most common cause of vision loss in people over age 40 and is the principal cause of blindness in the world.

Cholecystitis: Inflammation of the gallbladder.

Cholelythiasis: The presence of stones in the gallbladder.

Cirrhosis: A chronic disease of the liver marked by degeneration of cells, inflammation, and fibrous thickening of tissue.

Colitis: Inflammation of the lining of the colon.

Coronaroangiopathy: Angiopathy is the generic term for a disease of the blood vessels (arteries, veins, and capillaries). Coronary pertains to the arteries that surround and supply the heart.

Cysts: Cysts are fluid-filled sacs that occur in tissues in any part of the body.

Cystitis: Inflammation of the urinary bladder. It is often caused by infection and is usually accompanied by frequent, painful urination.

Diabetes Mellitus: A disease in which the body's ability to produce or respond to the hormone insulin is impaired, resulting in abnormal metabolism of carbohydrates and elevated levels of glucose in the blood and urine.

Diverticulosis: Diverticulosis is when pockets called diverticula form in the walls of the digestive tract. The inner layer of the intestine pushes through weak spots in the outer lining. This pressure makes them bulge out, making little pouches. Most often, it happens in the colon, the lower part of the large intestine.

Dyslipidemia: Refers to unhealthy levels of one or more kinds of lipid (fat) in the blood. Blood contains three main types of lipid: high-density lipoprotein (HDL) low-density lipoprotein (LDL) triglycerides.

Dyspeptic: Of or having indigestion.

-Ectomy: Signifying the surgical removal of a part of the body.

Encephalopathy: Disease, damage, or malfunction of the brain.

Endometritis: An inflammatory condition of the lining of the uterus, usually due to an infection.

Enteritis: Inflammation of the intestine, especially the small intestine.

Epigastric: Lying upon or over the stomach.

Erythrocytes: In medical terminology, erythro- means red, and -cyte means cell.

Essential tremor: A nerve disorder characterized by uncontrollable shaking, or tremors, in different parts and on different sides of the body. Areas affected often include the hands, arms, head, larynx, tongue, and chin.

Fibrocystosis: Characterized by the development of fibrous tissue and cystic spaces, typically in the pancreas or the breast.

Fibroma: A benign fibrous tumor of connective tissue.

Fibromyoma: A benign tumor derived from smooth muscle, most often of the uterus.

Gastroenterocolitis: Inflammation of the lining membrane of the stomach and the intestines characterized especially by nausea, vomiting, diarrhea, and cramps.

GFR: A test used to check how well the kidneys are working. Specifically, it estimates how much blood passes through the glomeruli each minute. Glomeruli are the tiny filters in the kidneys that filter waste from the blood.

Glaucoma: A condition of increased pressure within the eyeball, causing gradual loss of sight.

Glomeroneuropathy: Also known as glomerular nephritis is a term used to refer to several kidney diseases (usually affecting both kidneys).

Hashimoto's Disease: An autoimmune disease causing chronic inflammation and consequential failure of the thyroid gland.

Hematuria: The presence of blood in urine.

Hemorrhagic colitis: A type of gastroenteritis in which certain strains of the bacterium Escherichia coli infect the large intestine and produce a toxin (Shiga toxin) that causes bloody diarrhea and other serious complications.

Hepatitis: A disease characterized by inflammation of the liver.

Hepatomegaly: Abnormal enlargement of the liver.

Hepatosplenomegaly: The simultaneous enlargement of both the liver (hepatomegaly) and the spleen (splenomegaly).

Hernia: A condition in which part of an organ is displaced and protrudes through the wall of the containing cavity.

Hydronephrosis: Cystic distension of the kidney caused by the accumulation of urine in the renal pelvis due to obstruction of outflow and accompanied by atrophy of the kidney structure and cyst formation.

Hyperkeratosis: A thickening of the stratum corneum (the outermost layer of the epidermis).

Hyperthyroidism: A condition in which the thyroid gland produces too much of the hormone thyroxine. Hyperthyroidism can accelerate your body's metabolism significantly, causing sudden weight loss, a rapid or irregular heartbeat, sweating, and nervousness or irritability.

Hypertension: Abnormally high blood pressure

Renal Hypertension: Abnormally high blood pressure with renal etiology

Hypertonia: Increased tightness of muscle tone and reduced capacity of the muscle to stretch caused by damage to the motor nerve pathways in the central nervous system. Untreated hypertonia can lead to loss of function and deformity.

Hypertrophy: Enlargement or overgrowth of an organ or part of the body due to the increased size of the constituent cells.

Hypothyroidism: A disorder of the endocrine system in which the thyroid gland does not produce enough thyroid hormone. It can cause a number of symptoms, such as poor ability to tolerate cold, a feeling of tiredness, constipation, depression, and weight gain.

Hypotension: Abnormally low blood pressure.

Hypotonia: Decreased muscle tone and strength that results in floppiness.

Gastritis: Inflammation of the stomach.

Gastroenterocolitis: Inflammation of the lining membrane of the stomach and the intestines characterized especially by nausea, vomiting, diarrhea, and cramps.

Glomerulonephritis: Acute glomerulonephritis: one of a group of kidney diseases characterized by the abrupt onset of inflammation and proliferation of the glomeruli, microscopic structures within the kidney that are responsible for filtering the blood and producing urine.

Lacrimal channels: A small channel, the end of which is visible on the margin of each eyelid that drains the lacrimal (tear) fluid from the eye towards the lacrimal sac.

Leukocytes: White Blood Cells that help the body fight infections and other diseases.

Lipomatous nodes / Lipoma: A benign tumor of adipocytes (fat cells). Lipomas are common in the skin and are found anywhere on the body.

Lymphadenitis: Lymphadenitis is the inflammation of lymph nodes.

Medial meniscus: The medial meniscus of the knee is a thickened crescent-shaped cartilage pad between the two joints formed by the femur (the thigh bone) and the tibia (the shin bone).

Metrorrhagia: Uterine bleeding at irregular intervals, particularly between the expected menstrual periods. Metrorrhagia may be a sign of an underlying disorder, such as hormone imbalance, endometriosis, and uterine fibroids or, less commonly, cancer of the uterus.

Microcystosis: A condition in which red blood cells are unusually small as measured by their mean corpuscular volume.

Motor aphasia: The inability to speak or to organize the muscular movements of speech.

Myopia: The ability to see close objects more clearly than distant objects.

Nephritis: Inflammation of the kidney, which causes impaired kidney function. Nephritis can be due to a variety of causes, including kidney disease, autoimmune disease, and infection.

Nephrolithiasis: Kidney stone disease, a condition in which individuals form calculi (stones) within the renal pelvis and tubular lumens. Stones form from crystals that precipitate (separate) out of the urine.

Nephroscerosis: A progressive disease of the kidneys that results from sclerosis (hardening) of the small blood vessels in the kidneys.

Neuroses: A chronic disorder featuring irritability of the nervous system (nervousness) and characterized by anxiety and/or extreme behavior dedicated to avoid anxiety situations.

Osteoarthritis: A type of arthritis caused by inflammation, breakdown, and eventual loss of cartilage in the joints. Also known as degenerative arthritis.

Osteochondrosis: A disease that affects the progress of bone growth by killing bone tissue.

Parasitic liver cysts: Caused by infestation with the parasite Echinococcus granulosus. This parasite is found worldwide, but it is particularly common in areas of sheep and cattle farming. The adult tapeworm lives in the digestive tract of carnivores, such as dogs or wolves.

Phelbothrombosis: occurs when a blood clot (thrombosis) in a vein (phlebo) forms independently from the presence of inflammation of the vein (phlebitis).

Pleuritis: Inflammation of the pleura, which may be caused by infection, injury, or tumor. When the pleura becomes inflamed, it can produce more than the normal amount of fluid, causing a pleural effusion.

Pneumosclerosis: Excessive growth of connective tissue in the lungs as a result of various diseases.

Polyneuropathy: Damage or disease affecting peripheral nerves (peripheral neuropathy) in roughly the same areas on both sides of the body, featuring weakness, numbness, and burning pain.

Polypectomy: The removal of a polyp.

Prostatitis: Swelling and inflammation of the prostate gland, a walnut-sized gland situated directly below the bladder in men. The prostate gland produces fluid (semen) that nourishes and transports sperm. Prostatitis often causes painful or difficult urination.

Protenuria: Excess protein in the urine. The protein leaks through the kidney, most often through the glomeruli.

Ptosis: A drooping upper eyelid.

Quadriparalysis: A condition characterized by weakness in all four limbs (both arms and both legs).

Radiculopathy: Commonly referred to as pinched nerve, refers to a set of conditions in which one or more nerves are affected and do not work properly (a neuropathy). This can result in pain (radicular pain), weakness, numbness, or difficulty controlling specific muscles.

Retinal ablation: Removal of a segment of the eye's outer epithelial layer (Lasik surgery).

Retinoangiopathy: Damage to the eye due to high blood pressure.

Rheumatism: Any disease marked by inflammation and pain in the joints, muscles, or fibrous tissue, especially rheumatoid arthritis.

Rheumatoid arthritis: A chronic progressive disease causing inflammation in the joints and resulting in painful deformity and immobility, especially in the fingers, wrists, feet, and ankles.

Rheumatoid myocarditis: Heart muscle inflammation in a rheumatism.

Rhinosinitus: Also known as a sinus infection, is inflammation of the sinuses resulting in common symptoms like thick nasal mucus, a plugged nose, and pain in the face.

Steatosis hepatis: Non-alcoholic fatty liver disease.

Stenocardia: Contraction of the heart or its vessels due to a lack of oxygen, causing severe chest pain.

Struma: A swelling of the thyroid gland; a goiter.

Tachycardia: A relatively rapid heart action whether physiological (as after exercise) or pathological.

Transaminasis: Elevations in levels of the liver enzymes.

Uterine horn: The uterine horns are the points where the uterus and the fallopian tubes meet.

ABOUT THE AUTHOR

George Zdravkov was born and educated in Bulgaria. After attending the Medical University in Sofia, Bulgaria, he graduated as a medical doctor in 1986. Dr. Zdravkov completed his residency in neurology at the Medical University in Sofia, Bulgaria in 1997 and a specialization in radiology at the Medical Institute in Plodiv, Bulgaria in 1999. Fascinated by the diagnostic and curative possibilities offered by Traditional Chinese Medicine, he completed a specialization in acupuncture in 1988 at the Medical Academy in Sofia, Bulgaria. It was in Bulgaria that he participated in cutting-edge research and created innovative diagnostic techniques, publishing his findings in several books, while he was director of the Research Laboratory Apparatuses and Systems for Energy-Information Exchange at the Technical University in Plovdiv, Bulgaria.

After coming to the United States, Dr. Zdravkov continued his research while completing a specialization in Electro-neuro diagnostics in 2001 at the East-West University in Chicago, IL. Dr. Zdravkov additionally completed a specialization in Acupuncture and Oriental Medicine in 2004 at Midwest College of Oriental Medicine in Racine, Wisconsin, and a specialization in Acupuncture and TCM, in 2014 at the Shanghai International Acupuncture Training Center in Shanghai, China, as well as the International Structural Acupuncture Course for Physicians: A Palpation Based Approach, between 2014- 2015 at Harvard Medical School in Cambridge, MA.

During this time, Dr. Zdravkov developed a thriving medical practice at the Center for Integrative Medicine in Park Ridge, IL. (www.integralmed.us)

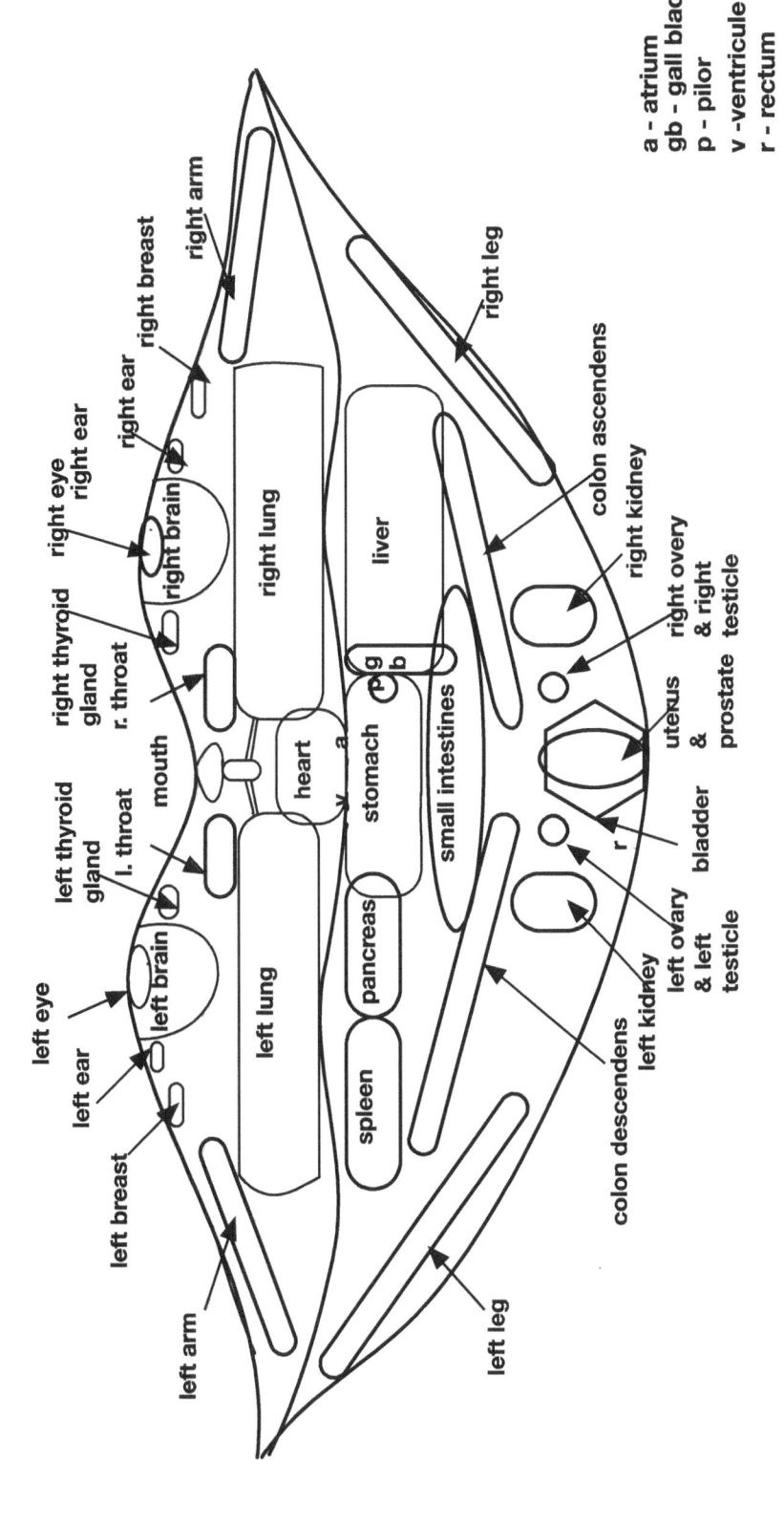

www.ingramcontent.com/pod-product-compliance
Lightning Source LLC
Chambersburg PA
CBHW051146220526
45473CB00003B/679